HOMEOPATHY AND
AUTISM SPECTRUM DISORDER

of related interest

**Understanding Controversial Therapies
for Children with Autism, Attention Deficit
Disorder, and Other Learning Disabilities**
A Guide to Complementary and Alternative Medicine
Lisa A. Kurtz
ISBN 978 1 84310 864 1
eISBN 978 1 84642 761 9
Part of the JKP Essentials series

A Brief Guide to Autism Treatments
Elisabeth Hollister Sandberg and Becky L. Spritz
ISBN 978 1 84905 904 6
eISBN 978 0 85700 650 9

HOMEOPATHY AND
AUTISM SPECTRUM DISORDER

A GUIDE FOR PRACTITIONERS
AND FAMILIES

MIKE ANDREWS

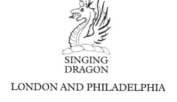

SINGING
DRAGON

LONDON AND PHILADELPHIA

First published in 2014
by Singing Dragon
an imprint of Jessica Kingsley Publishers
73 Collier Street
London N1 9BE, UK
and
400 Market Street, Suite 400
Philadelphia, PA 19106, USA

www.singingdragon.com

Library of Congress Cataloging in Publication Data
Andrews, Mike, 1959-
  Homeopathy and autism spectrum disorder : a guide for
practitioners and families / Mike Andrews.
     pages cm
  Includes bibliographical references and index.
  ISBN 978-1-84819-168-6 (alk. paper)
  1. Autism spectrum disorders–Homeopathic treatment. I. Title.
  RC553.A88A454 2014
  616.85'88206–dc23
                                2014004225

British Library Cataloguing in Publication Data
A CIP catalogue record for this book is available from the British Library

ISBN 978 1 84819 168 6
eISBN 978 0 85701 128 2

Printed and bound in Great Britain

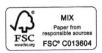

I dedicate this book to my parents, Bryan and Jean, who gave me the freedom to follow my own path in life. To my wife, Judy, for her unstinting love and support, and to my colleagues for their friendship and learning together.

ACKNOWLEDGEMENTS

Thank you to my proofreaders, Judy Andrews and Jane Wood. To all the homeopaths who have taken time to talk to me and especially all of those that have contributed to the book.

Thanks also go to Bethany Gower, Lisa Clark and Sarah Minty at Jessica Kingsley Publishers, for their advice and patience.

DISCLAIMER

The information in this book is intended for information purposes only. It is not a substitute for professional medical advice, nor to be used for purposes of self-diagnosis or self-treatment.

Homeopathic treatments should only ever be taken under the direct guidance and care of a properly and fully trained homeopathic practitioner.

Neither the publishers nor author will accept any responsibility for any ill effects resulting from the use or misuse of the information contained in this book.

CONTENTS

PREFACE

This book will benefit several different groups of people in different ways.

If you are a parent of or carer for a child on the autism spectrum this book will give you the confidence to try homeopathy for your child. You will be able to start the homeopathic therapeutic journey with clear expectations of homeopathy and what might be achievable for your child. You will gain an understanding of what homeopathy is and how it works.

There are several other books previously published, which are collections of 'cured' cases and these are well worth reading too; however in this book I have tried to look at what is being achieved in different parts of the world and by different practitioners on a larger scale.

This is not a book about self-treatment or remedies to try for your child; but it does explain the different types of approaches that homeopaths around the world are using and how successful they are. It also empowers you to ask questions of a homeopath that you might be considering working with, and looks at what the homeopath might expect of you! Homeopathy is not a quick fix; it is something that you will need to commit to for the long haul, nevertheless I hope that this book will give you the confidence to explore this approach to helping your child.

If you are a healthcare professional or teacher working with children on the autism spectrum, the book will give you an understanding of the journey that your clients are undertaking using homeopathic treatment. It should give you the confidence to suggest to families you are working with that they might like to consider homeopathic treatment.

If you are a practising homeopath or homeopathic student this book will give you a good overview of the different methodologies being used worldwide and the type of results that they are achieving. It will make it easier for you to repertorise your cases and to understand the remedies that are often indicated. It will give you a sense of what you are likely to achieve with the clients you work with and a good understanding of autism spectrum disorders (ASD) and some of the other treatments that patients might be using.

The book primarily focuses on working with children with ASD. There have been cases reported (Elia 2012) where homeopathy has helped adults on the spectrum and also cases with teenagers (Ron 2013; see also pp.88–89). However, in treating any condition it is always better to start as early as possible when symptoms are first noticed. Patterns of health and behaviour become more concretised with the passage of time and thus harder to shift. In practice the author, and many other homeopaths, are often called on to commence treatment with children in the age range seven to ten and achieve great benefits for those children, in terms of reduction of aggression and improved general health.

The autism spectrum is vast: from cases of high functioning autism (formerly known as Asperger's), to severe autism accompanied by fits and brain damage, from no speech to taciturn to loquacious, from mild to violent; yet homeopathy can benefit all of these groups. However, we still do not yet fully understand why some cases benefit more than others, regardless of the depth of the diagnosis.

Homeopathy, like a number of other complementary or alternative systems of healthcare is truly holistic. The holistic approach takes account of all of the system in which the patient lives; parental influences from pre-conception to pregnancy and beyond, to the ancestral or genetic health patterns running through a family; as well as a child's physical, mental and emotional symptoms. To determine the most appropriate homeopathic remedy to prescribe, dreams or specific fears are of equal value alongside the child's specific food likes or dislikes, their allergies or their persistently enlarged tonsils.

Homeopathy is a form of holistic medicine based on the principle that like treats like, the Greek meaning of the word 'homoeopathy' is 'similar suffering'. This was the original name given to this system of medicine by its founder Hahnemann over two hundred years ago. 'Homeopathy' is an American spelling of the word and has been adopted on the internet, so is now replacing the former spelling.

Homeopathic medicines are made from specially prepared highly diluted substances and prescriptions are tailored to each individual patient, according to their specific symptoms. Homeopaths treat the person as a whole rather than the disease or diagnosis per se. Homeopaths regard all the symptoms of a patient's condition – mental, emotional and physical – as evidence of an inner disturbance and seek to return the patient to a state of balance based on these signs and characteristics.

Homeopathy has much to offer the child, or adult, with a diagnosis on the autism spectrum and I hope that you will be inspired by the information in this book.

CHAPTER ONE

CAN MORE BE DONE TO TREAT AUTISM SPECTRUM DISORDER?

Limitations of behaviour modification, nutritional therapy and biomedicine and other approaches which do not utilise the integrated approach of homeopathy. The potential of homeopathic treatment.

Professionals working in the field of Autism Spectrum Disorder (ASD) and parents or carers will be aware of and perhaps have used many different therapies and approaches to help the child with ASD. My area of specialisation is homeopathic medicine, so these are my personal insights having worked in the field of natural health for nearly 25 years, as well as researching the published work of other homeopaths and talking to many colleagues.

A homeopath tries to get to the cause of a problem rather than to mask or modify symptoms. As that wonderful quote by the 15th-century philosopher Paracelsus (1493–1541) so succinctly puts it:

> Those who merely study and treat the effects of disease are like those who imagine that they can drive away the winter by brushing the snow from the door. It is not the snow that causes the winter, but the winter that causes the snow.
>
> (Paracelsus in Hartmann 1998, p.255)

Autism charities such as Research Autism and Autism Research Institute provide an enormous amount of information and have evaluated the effectiveness of different approaches as much as is possible.

The truly holistic approach of homeopathy is one of the few therapeutic interventions that sees physical, mental and emotional aspects of the child, or adult, being treated as equally important. All of these are integrated into the case history, subsequent treatment plan and evaluation. Homeopathy treats each case individually rather than according to a pre-set protocol and as Paracelsus explains, looks for the causative factors rather than attempting to manage or suppress symptoms.

Research Autism (2013) reports that the most commonly used interventions used in the UK include:

- diets, such as the gluten-free, casein-free diet

- behavioural approaches, such as the Lovaas method

- medication, such as anti-psychotics

- augmentative communication, such as the Picture Exchange Communication System (PECS)

- sensory integration techniques

- specialist education, e.g. schools for children with autism

- speech and language therapy.

BEHAVIOUR MODIFICATION

The use and provision of therapeutic interventions obviously varies from country to country, some are available privately and some are state provided. Therapies will vary in the depth of their work; a number will be aimed at teaching parenting strategies to manage behaviour in an acceptable manner, others will be teaching the child techniques to help them to manage their environment better. Approaches used might include: Applied Behavioural Analysis (ABA), treatments for sensory-processing disorders, Treatment and Education of Autistic and Related Communication Handicapped Children (TEACCH), developmental and educational approaches, speech therapy might also include behavioural considerations. ABA remains a controversial approach and the hours needed to carry out a full programme could further stress an already challenged family. The cost of long term intensive one-to-one therapy is another factor to be considered.

There is, it seems, the potential to suppress or repress aspects of the whole homeostatic system, which aims to maintain balance within the individual; and this could potentially lead to additional or new problems, either physical or psychological. It is important to find ways to assist and enable the child on the autism spectrum to integrate into society, on their terms.

One of the key points that Attwood (2003) makes in his DVD series is that it is the 'neuronormal' who have to improve their understanding of the world of the ASD child or adult. The significance of this, both educationally, and in the way that parents communicate to their children cannot be underestimated. Adjusting teaching methods to the needs of the individual is so important and unfortunately often neglected.

CONVENTIONAL PHARMACEUTICAL DRUGS
The Charter of Rights for Persons with Autism number 18 (European Parliament 1996) enshrines the right of people with autism to freedom from pharmaceutical abuse or misuse.

> Except for short periods of time and in particular circumstances, the use of major tranquilisers cannot be justified. Certain atypical tranquilisers, used at low dosages, may be appropriate for certain individuals on a longer term basis. Generally the use of tranquilisers does nothing to help the basic autism but serves only to sedate the afflicted person and to make him or her more manageable. At the same time such drugs will impair learning and decrease the happiness and understanding of the individual. Long term effects, including the occurrence of Tardive dyskinesias are irreversible. (p.2)

However, talking to any group of parents of children with an ASD diagnosis a large number will be found to be on medications of various kinds. As Shattock, Waltz and Whiteley (2004 p.2) state 'medication tends to be used against specific target symptoms such as epilepsy, hyperactivity and stereotypic behaviours rather than targeting core autistic features'. As later chapters will show, homeopathy has the potential to address core features of autism and is without side-effects.

Neuroleptic drugs originally developed for treating schizophrenia have been used as a liquid cosh to calm people down and make them easier to manage. Shattock *et al.* (2004, p.5) in their excellent paper 'The Use of Medication for People with Autism Spectrum Disorders' state that in patients taking the drugs Risperidone, Olanzepine and Quatiepine 'there have been substantial and unacceptable weight gains in people, with ASD, using these medications and there may be a heightened risk of development of diabetes' (p.5).

Antidepressants such as the commonly prescribed selective serotonin reuptake inhibitors (SSRIs) have well known side-effects and have not been tested on children. Concerns have been raised about the increased suicidal tendencies associated with these drugs.

Stimulant medication such as Ritalin is more commonly considered a drug for children with Attention Deficit Hyperactivity Disorder (ADHD) or Attention Deficit Disorder (ADD), but many children with ASD will have been previously mis-diagnosed as ADHD or ADD or have a dual diagnosis.

Obviously there are complex clinical decisions to be made about these medications and their effect, not just on the quality of life of the patient, but also on the wider family and school community. If your child is taking prescribed medication and then for whatever reason you wish to change the dosage, you must discuss this with the prescribing physician.

DIETARY APPROACHES

The line between biomedicine and dietary approaches can be blurred, but for the sake of this book I am defining biomedicine as the application of the principles of biology and physiology to clinical medicine; and dietary approaches as the inclusion or exclusion of certain foods in the diet. If the system is already overloaded, as it often seems to be in patients with ASD, it seems to make sense not to add to that load by avoiding the following types of food: packaged processed foods, foods containing artificial sweeteners, white flour, white sugar, pesticides, colour additives, flavour enhancers or preservatives. In essence removing all artificial additives, colourings and highly processed foods. The use of microwaves or plastic packaging and storage can also be a problem for some children.

The following should be added to the diet: fresh organic foods, filtered water, and some basic food supplements.

In addition to exclusion diets some people may be using the following supplements: vitamin C, zinc, vitamin B6, Omega-3 fatty acids, magnesium and many others; probiotics may also be used to improve gastrointestinal function. It is important to speak to a suitability qualified practitioner to check the optimum dosages of any of these basic supplements.

Although these approaches can be helpful, the drawback is that they deal with effects rather than causes. Factors that mitigate against dietary and other nutritional approaches in the treatment of ASD include the problem of compliance; mealtimes can be a battleground in many families and imposing a restrictive diet on one family member can add extra tensions as well as problems with peers. It can be difficult to eat out or away from home and this adds to perceptions of the child being odd. As the child becomes older, the parents have far less control over what their child eats. The long-term use of high-quality supplements can be costly. Nevertheless there is certainly plenty of anecdotal evidence to suggest that these diets do help some children (Whiteley and Shattock 2002).

> Peptides with opioid activity derived from dietary sources, in particular, foods that contain gluten and casein, pass through an abnormally permeable intestinal membrane and enter the central nervous system to exert an effect on neurotransmission, as well as producing other physiologically-based symptoms. Numerous parents and professionals worldwide have found that removal of these exogenously derived compounds

through exclusion diets can produce some amelioration in autistic and related behaviours.

And

The opioid-excess hypothesis of autism suggests that autism is the consequence of the incomplete breakdown and excessive absorption of peptides with opioid activity (derived from foods which contain gluten and casein), causing disruption to biochemical and neuroregulatory processes. Biochemical evidence has indicated the presence of increased levels of peptides in the urine of people with autism, and previous behavioural studies have demonstrated a connection between the long term exclusion of gluten and casein from the diet and improvement in the behaviour of some children with autism. (Whiteley 1999 p.45)

I would argue that opioid excess is a symptom of rather than the causative factor of autism as seems to be stated here: *why do autistic individuals have this problem?*

The theory behind the gluten-free/casein-free diet is that undigested casein and gluten peptides leak into the bloodstream and then circulate to the brain, causing opiate-like effects – such as vagueness, disorientation, painlessness and other possible behavioural changes. Foods containing gluten are foods containing, barley, oats, rye and wheat in whatever form. Foods containing casein are cow or goat dairy products such as milk, cheese, butter, cream, yogurt and infant formulas. Anyone who has tried to follow this diet will know how carefully food labels have to be read, as both gluten and casein may be hidden ingredients in many processed foods, seasonings and drinks. Other diets include the Specific Carbohydrate Diet, the Stone Age diet and the Gut and Psychology Syndrome diet (GAPS).

My initial recommendation would be to look at the Feingold Diet, as this is the diet that more of my clients have found helpful and is less difficult to follow than the gluten-free/casein-free diet. There has been some positive research about the Feingold Diet, which requires the individual to avoid some additives, such as synthetic colourings, flavourings and preservatives, as well as salicylate, a natural plant toxin found in some foodstuffs and medicines. The majority of families who use the Feingold Diet do so to help a family member with behaviour and/or learning problems. The supporters of the Feingold Diet believe that it can be used to treat a wide range of problems, including some of those faced by people with autism.

The Feingold Diet is based on the premise that allergic reactions or sensitivities to certain types of foods cause or contribute to ADD/ADHD symptoms, such as hyperactivity, impulsive and compulsive behaviour, short attention span, neuro-muscular difficulties, cognitive and perceptual disturbances, sleep problems and so on (Feingold Association, 2014). Many ADD/ADHD sufferers who follow the Feingold programme have experienced great improvements in focus and behaviour. There is apparently considerable research to back this up and studies in the early 1990s show that around 75 per cent of children improve on a diet that restricts additives. Autism Research Institute (2009) reported that 58 per cent of 899 families who had tried the Feingold diet found that it was helpful for their child.

HOW HOMEOPATHY AND BIOMEDICINE DIFFER

Fran Sheffield (2008) in her excellent article, 'Homeopathy and the treatment of autism spectrum disorders (part two)' comments on and compares homeopathy and biomedicine as follows:

> **Homeopathy** is a simple and unchanging system of medicine. Its therapeutic action comes from the consistent application of a natural law, the law of similars.

> **Biomedicine** is a conglomerate of complex and changing treatments that vary from practitioner to practitioner, and from year to year. It has no underpinning law to guide practice.

> **Homeopathy** is safe. It has no toxic side-effects and will not interact with other prescribed substances. It does no harm.

Biomedicine is capable of toxic side-effects, leaching of vital minerals, and detrimental interactions with other substances. It can and does harm.

Homeopathy is based on the observation that an illness or disease can be removed by the short lived effects of a sufficiently similar second disease of either natural or medicinal origin. Once free of the short lived effects of the second disease, and no longer suffering from the original disease, the body returns to a state of independent health and homeostasis. Biochemical pathways are restored and pathogens die out uneventfully.

Biomedicine is based on an assumption that the body's biochemistry, or a pathogen affecting it, contains the causes, rather than the intermediate effects of, ill health. It therefore uses chemicals to suppress or control symptoms, force a particular response, or kill the pathogens. Side-effects, overgrowths, and die-off symptoms are common.

Homeopathy treats simply and methodically. A single medicine is prescribed according to the presenting symptom complex and the law of similars. Each dose is observed for the type of response it triggers in the unwell person. An improvement followed by a partial return of the original symptoms requires a further dose of the same remedy; an improvement followed by the emergence of new symptoms requires a dose of a newly matching remedy; and so on. In this way, the practitioner moves the patient step by step toward perfect health.

Biomedicine treatment takes place in cumulative and increasingly complex layers. Medicines are prescribed for their suppressive or palliate effects in opposition to single symptoms. The use of medicines to stimulate rather than suppress the body's own recuperative efforts is unknown in biomedicine.

Homeopathy does not create resistant pathogens or increase food intolerances.

Biomedicine treatment of pathogens with antibiotics and anti-fungals can lead to re-colonisation by more resistant forms. Severe dietary restrictions may increase rather than reduce food intolerances.

Homeopathy compliance is easy. There are no complicated dosage regimes or drastic diets. Homoeopathic medicines are pleasant tasting, and doses are small; they are well-tolerated by children.

Biomedicine compliance can be difficult. Medicines may taste unpleasant or be difficult to swallow. Dietary restrictions can turn meal times into battles, and complicated treatment regimes disturb sleep and disrupt family life.

Homeopathic treatment is relatively inexpensive. Consultation fees vary between practitioners, but once treatment has been established, consultations are usually weeks to months apart. Expensive and extensive investigations are not needed, and medicinal costs are low.

Biomedical costs are expensive. Consultation fees vary between practitioners; plans for extended treatment requiring costly investigations and tests, followed by multiple medicines and treatments, are the norm.

Homeopathy can frequently improve on biomedical treatment.

Biomedical treatment does not seem to add to improvements produced by good homeopathic prescriptions.

Homeopathy when applied according to sound principles has been shown to bring improvement for the great majority of children, and often rapidly.

Biomedical treatment is slow and demanding on parents and children. Results are variable. While some children improve, a significant number, 50 per cent or more, are not helped by many of its approaches, and some regress during treatment (Sheffield 2008, p.18).

MAKING THE TRANSITION FROM BIOMEDICINE TO HOMEOPATHY – FRAN SHEFFIELD (2008)

Biomedical dependency

In an ideal world, parents would suspend most, if not all, biomedical interventions when commencing homeopathic treatment. Case management would then be clearer and less complex for both practitioner and patient. In reality, this rarely happens. Initially, most parents remain highly dependent on biomedical treatments until their confidence in homeopathy has grown. Only then is it possible for them to consider discontinuing some or all of its interventions. Reasons for this dependence include the following:

Biomedicine's sophisticated and impressive appearance

Biomedicine treatments are complex, expensive, and embraced by highly educated doctors, paediatricians, specialists, and allied therapists. In contrast, homeopathy, with its infrequent water doses or sugar pills prescribed by a limited number of professional homoeopaths, appears too subtle or gentle in the eyes of some to achieve the improvements promised by biomedicine. For this reason, parents can easily attribute the gains from homeopathic treatment to rigorous simultaneous biomedical treatment.

Fear

Parents trying to 'recover' their ASD-affected children are frequently dealing with:

- Fear of missing the window period of early childhood in which biomedicine has the potential to make the greatest difference.

- Fear that valuable gains will be lost if their child regresses because biomedicine was suspended in favour of an unknown homeopathy.

- Fear of offending professionals who may currently be helping their child.

- Fear of being without the support, understanding, and friendship of a biomedical community when much of society still struggles to understand or accept their child's confronting behaviours.

- Fear that aggravations arising from homeopathic treatment (or high doses of the supplements or medicines that become unnecessary with successful treatment) may really be the reactivation of gut dysbiosis or a sign of regression.

Misidentification of homeopathy

Homeopathy is generally understood poorly and represented inaccurately by biomedical proponents and on biomedical forums. It is often wrongly identified as the use of nosodes, isodes, human symbiodes, or complexes, used in a 'this for that' manner, or as a series of routine remedies prescribed according to a causal history. Parents whose children have been treated in this inadequate manner (by homeopathic and non-homeopathic practitioners) have a limited appreciation of homeopathy and report variable results. As a consequence, seasoned members of biomedical forums generally advise that, while homeopathy is sometimes helpful, it is also unreliable; and that its practitioners usually know too little of ASD issues or biomedical treatments for parents to entrust them with the complete care of their child.

Prior investment

Biomedicine is a field in which the ground rules are still being laid, and it is not unusual to find highly motivated parents who are better informed about biomedical treatment options and expected responses than many professionals. These parents are often solely responsible for their child's biomedical treatment, and because of their experience in this area, may be sought out by newer or less-knowledgeable parents for the information they can share – something that is obviously flattering and gratifying. In other instances, parents may confuse any success from their child's biomedical treatment with their own success as parents. Either way, a lot more than time and money may be invested by parents in their children's biomedical treatment than is likely with homeopathy.

Assisting in the transition

Short of refusing to accept a child for treatment, the best course of action for the homeopath is to address the above issues with time, patience, education, and a preparedness to support parents in the difficult transition from an allopathic to a homeopathic mode of treatment. If homeopathy's potential is to be fully realised by countless numbers of ASD affected children, then we as practitioners also have to present clear, accurate, and consistent information on its principles and practice to the biomedical community. Now, that's a challenge worth picking up. (Sheffield 2008, p.20)

CHELATION

The most aggressive biomedical intervention is the detoxification and chelation of heavy toxic metals. It would certainly be worth exploring the far gentler path of homeopathic detoxification if it was felt that this was necessary. Amy Lansky (2005 podcast) thinks that with the 'right remedy in most cases the body will naturally chelate'.

THE CANDIDA PROBLEM

The anti-Candida diet restricts sugars and refined carbohydrates to control Candida overgrowth, which has effects on brain gut dysbiosis. It is thus seen as an important tool in the biomedical armoury. Fran Sheffield (2008), an Australian homeopath writes about some of the problems she perceives with this diet. In Chapter four, I have included a long article from the Israeli homeopath, Danny Dushan

Ron, about his approach and successes with homeopathic treatment against Candida, an approach definitely worth exploring alongside more conventional homeopathic treatment. Using this approach may have the advantage over the conventional approach to Candida, as problems of 'die off' and re-colonisation might be avoided.

IN CONCLUSION

It is important that homeopaths working with ASD patients are aware of the range of different biomedical treatments and diets as many parents will be already using or considering these therapies for their children and as Sheffield (2008) states, homeopaths' lack of knowledge about biomedicine can be a reason why parents on internet forums have been unwilling to entrust homeopaths with their care.

Carol Boyce (2010), in her excellent article, 'Lost generation: the rise and rise of regressive autism', argues that managing a protocol including a gluten-free/dairy-free diet, chelation for heavy metal toxicity, anti-fungal medications for candidiasis and other nutritional supplements is difficult with small children, stressful for parents and child and very expensive to maintain. She says that:

> Parents and practitioners describe a plateau effect, where the child makes initial rapid progress once on the diet and then again with the supplementation, but gradually progress stalls, and falls short of the progress necessary for a re-diagnosis of neurotypical. It is at this stage that Defeat Autism Now (DAN) families look for other options and might consider homeopathy. (p.18)

Boyce goes on to write that 'If we consider ASD to be a neurological expression of a metabolic problem, then homeopathy is a logical choice for such cases' (p.18).

Later chapters will explore the clinical results and methodologies that homeopaths are using in the treatment of ASD. Boyce suggests that:

> We can initially take the pressure off the system by removing the maintaining causes – gluten and casein – from the diet and supplementation to address the nutritional deficiencies that impact the ability to synthesise, catabolise and excrete. Ultimately, though, the body must be able to complete these processes independently in order to sustain health in the absence of supplementation. Once the metabolic processes are reset and working efficiently, it stands to reason that external supplementation is no longer required and has the potential to overload the system, especially a system that has already had problems with excretion and subsequent toxicity. (p.19)

From the homeopathic perspective biomedical treatments are palliating or suppressing symptoms rather than addressing the underlying causes of an out-of-balance holistic system and intrinsic errors of metabolism. However the value of biomedicine cannot be underestimated in all that it has achieved for so many ASD sufferers; and a judicious combination of biomedicine and homeopathy has the potential to achieve deeper and more long lasting improvements.

The same question has also been asked by Research Autism (2013) – what are interventions supposed to do?:

> increase adaptive behaviours, such as social skills, communication skills or imaginative behaviours; reduce or eliminate problematic behaviours, such as self-harm or aggression towards others; treat co-existing conditions, such as epilepsy or gastro-intestinal problems. Improve or enhance the quality of life of the person with autism.

It is my experience, and that of many other homeopaths around the world, that homeopathy can do all of these things. It is my aim to share the results of my experience and research over the next few chapters.

CHAPTER TWO

WHAT IS ASD?

*Overview of diagnosis. Causative factors — genetics,
exposure to toxins both environmental and medical.
What is happening from a homeopathic perspective?*

OVERVIEW OF DIAGNOSIS

The Diagnostic Statistical Manual (DSM-5 2013), describes autism spectrum disorder (ASD) as a neurodevelopmental disorder with three severity levels. Level 1 represents the highest functioning end of the spectrum and presents similarly to the condition previously diagnosed as Asperger's syndrome. Level 3 denotes the lowest functioning end of the spectrum and involves very severe communication impairments and extremely restricted behaviours.

The borders between these diagnosis levels can sometimes be hazy and it is beyond the scope of this book to go into classification of diagnosis. However it can be both useful and important to take the diagnosis into account so as to be clear as to possible treatment outcomes.

There may be intellectual impairment and autism together, increasing the likelihood of aggression, destruction of property and increased tantrums. Autism and intellectual impairment (previously called mental retardation) are not necessarily present in all cases but there may be a joint diagnosis.

There can also be a joint diagnosis of Attention Deficit and Hyperactivity Disorder (ADHD) or Attention Deficit Disorder (ADD), indeed many ASD children have been formally or mis-diagnosed with ADHD or ADD. As with any child or adult in the general population they may also have a range of other physical health problems.

In the United States it is estimated that between 1 in 50 or 1 in 88 children have ASD; 695,000 people in the United Kingdom. There is a problem in verifying exact numbers as figures are not collated in each country and there is debate as to whether the conditions are under- or over-diagnosed; however the increased prevalence of all diagnoses on the spectrum is surely, and sadly, without doubt. Many countries worldwide report a growing number of cases including India, where there are an estimated six million people with autism (Gupta *et al.* 2010), and Kenya; 2.64 per cent of South Korean children aged 7–12 have ASD (Kim 2011). Aspect (Autism Spectrum Disorder 2013), the Australian autism service provider, estimates that there are 230,000 Australians living with ASD. Autism is no respecter of borders or cultures and is a worldwide epidemic, although there are certain cultural groups where numbers are higher or lower. The Somali refugee population in the UK has particularly high rates of ASD, while the Amish community in the US has lower ASD rates than the larger population.

Children and adults diagnosed with ASD have delays or abnormal functioning in the following areas:

1. Social interaction/impaired social ability:

    - unusual nonverbal behaviour such as lack of eye contact, facial expression, gestures

    - failure to develop peer relationships, difficulties sharing with others

    - lack of social or emotional response

    - difficulty in recognising and understanding another person's feelings or perspective.

2. Language and social communication:

    - delayed or lack of development of spoken language

    - difficulty in sustaining or initiating conversation

    - repetitive use of language, words and phrases, e.g. echolalia

- lack of varied or spontaneous play
- flat or high-pitched speech
- narrow bands of passionate interests or obsessions
- difficulty in comprehension
- preference for activities that require little verbal interaction.

3. Behaviours, sensory or motor functions:

- restricted, repetitive, ritualised and stereotyped patterns of behaviour and activity
- awkwardness or delayed development of fine and gross motor skills
- hyper- or hypo-sensitivity to pain, light, sound, crowds and other external stimuli
- inflexible behaviour and difficulty in coping with change.

CAUSATIVE FACTORS – GENETICS, EXPOSURE TO TOXINS BOTH ENVIRONMENTAL AND MEDICAL

Although genetic factors are part of the story, it seems improbable that rates of autism would have risen so rapidly in recent years if genetics were the only factor. Like many contemporary diseases, the causes of autism are likely to be multi-factorial.

There are many chemical and environmental assaults upon any child born into the world today, both internal and external, the long-term effects of which are not really known. We, and our children, are exposed to many toxins such as fluorocarbons; heavy metals; ingredients in cosmetics and toiletries; insecticide, pesticide and herbicide residues in food; processed foods and so on. The increasing number of immunisations exposes the body to aluminium, mercury and other toxins. While food sensitivities play their part in the expression and severity of ASD symptoms, I see these as a symptom of an already damaged system rather than as a causative factor per se. The effects of factors such as IVF (Halladay 2013) and fertility drugs, maternal fever in pregnancy and parental exposure to environmental pollutants have all been suggested as possible causes of autism. However, as with most research into the causes of autism, there is research for and against most factors.

Whatever the causes, it does not help to feel guilty or blame yourself for your child's current health as all of us prefer to act on the best information available to us at the time. As a homeopath, I do not feel that it is my job to campaign or to speculate as to the possible causes of the child's ASD diagnosis, but rather to look for the changes in disposition and the symptoms expressed by the child and to prescribe on the basis of the symptom picture presented, so helping them to achieve their maximum potential.

Although many people implicate the current immunisation programme in the rise of autism, there are cases of autism where the child has not been immunised and if that were the single factor, surely we would all be on the autism spectrum. Although there seem to be countless cases where children's health has changed dramatically after an immunisation, just because two things happen together doesn't mean one has caused the other – this is the difference between association and causality. If all children are immunised around the age when autism is usually first detected, this does not necessary demonstrate a causative link between the two events. There have, however, still been several court cases around the world where immunisation has been implicated in a child's developmental changes. It might be useful to remember that it is not just the current exposure to vaccines and their adjuncts but now several generations' exposure which need to be taken into account.

The environmental factor would seem to be indicated when the child develops normally and then regresses: but there may be a trigger to latent genetic factors. It is also possible that the child born with ASD has been exposed to environmental toxins in utero. Social and educational pressures may also have a role to play in the increase of ASD.

WHAT IS GOING ON HOMEOPATHICALLY?

One of the fundamental principles upon which homeopathic philosophy is based is the principle of susceptibility. Why it is that one person will react to a substance or pathogen in the environment and another person will not? By taking a full in-depth case history the homeopath seeks to understand the individual's in-born and acquired sensitivities and to strengthen the body's energy system.

If there is an obvious causative factor, it can be necessary to prescribe isopathically or on the basis of 'never been well since'.

The founder of the homeopathic system of medicine, Samuel Hahnemann (1842), states the philosophy on which homeopathic treatment is based clearly in his book *The Organon of Medicine* (translated 1921) in aphorism 211:

> the state of the disposition of the patient often chiefly determines the selection of the homeopathic remedy; as being a decidedly characteristic symptom which can least of all remain concealed from the accurately observing physician. (p.233)

By disposition he means the characteristic symptoms of the patient, mental and emotional, physical likes and dislikes, and so on which mark out one individual from another.

He suggests, in aphorism 212 (p.233) that a 'powerful medicinal substance [will] notably alter the state of the disposition and mind in the healthy individual who tests it and every medicine does so in a different manner'.

The homeopath's task is to match the 'disposition' of a patient with the changes previously observed in those testing the medicinal substance, as Hahnemann (1842, 1921) writes in aphorism 213:

> we shall therefore never be able to cure…homoeopathically… if we do not observe…symptoms…relating to the changes in the state of mind and disposition, and if we do not select for the patient's relief, from among the medicines…is also capable of producing a similar state of the disposition and mind. (pp.233–234)

You will see that this is not a simple 'doctrine of signatures', but a far more complex analysis based on the principle of 'like treats like', *similia similibus curentur*, and homeopathy itself means 'like suffering'.

In a state of health the body produces a reaction to the disease in order to overcome it, however the disease is sometimes too powerful for the body to overcome, this results in either chronic or re-occurring ill health or morbidity. The homeopathic prescription is aimed to work with the body's own defence mechanism to overcome the disease. In a healthy state the body is able to respond to negative influences, but when we enter into a permanent state of ill health or disease the body becomes stuck in its reaction. The idea of homeopathic treatment is that by treating like with like we give the body the information it needs to respond to the problem and swing back to health. The speed at which this happens will depend on the depth of the disease and any physical damage which has already occurred.

There may also be what homeopaths refer to as maintaining causes; that is, continuing exposure to aggravating factors which overload the body's ability to respond. In the case of ASD these might be specifically poor gut health or heavy metal toxicity; although a well-chosen remedy can at times address this on its own without the need for other changes.

In some respects it could be postulated that the genetic viability or vitality of the human race is declining and certainly within homeopathic thinking the family medical history and heredity has always been taken into account in prescribing for children. This area of homeopathic treatment is known as 'miasmatic treatment'. Traditionally this might be looked at as inherited tendencies to under-function (Psora), tendencies to excess or over-production (Sycotic), tendency to destructive processes (Syphilitic), tendency to burn out, 'consumptive' (Tubercular), tendency to overstretch (Carcinogenic). There is no doubt from looking at the range of the most commonly prescribed remedies by homeopaths from around the world for ASD that *Medorrhinum, Tuberculinum, Carcinosin* and *Mercurius* are among the most commonly prescribed remedies for ASD and these are key remedies that help to clear the miasms or inherited factors. (This is something of a simplification as all homeopathic remedies are classified according to their miasmatic influence.)

As stated earlier, there is much debate within the field of conventional medicine as to the causes of ASD and although there is a genetic background, this does not explain the rapid increase in the disease. If genetics is the cause, one also has to take into account the developing field of epigenetics – that there are factors which turn genes on and off. Genetics alone cannot explain the great increase in autism over recent years. The eminent homeopath, Dr. Luc de Schepper (2011) finds that in his experience:

> the most neglected factor in the ASD epidemic is (an internal emotional factor) as the accent in allopathy [conventional medicine] is on external factors (environment) and heredity.

and

> as in any development of any disease the emotional, mental and physical triggers are important and cannot be neglected. All of them will be able as indicated in epigenetics to silence certain genes during the stages of the development of the foetus.

He thinks that the pregnancy story and family medical history are of enormous importance. I feel that perhaps he overemphasises the 'internal emotional factor' as upsets during pregnancy are nothing new, what is new is the exposure to so many toxins both in the form of medicines and environment. We also have to consider the effects of suppression of many disease processes by conventional medicine and whether this could be a factor. The allopathic/conventional approach treats on the basis of opposites, whereas homeopathy treats on the basis of similars. If you are suffering with nausea for example, conventional medicine will prescribe an anti-sickness drug to stop the body's reaction. Whereas the homeopath will prescribe a remedy which is capable of producing sickness thus enabling the body to overcome the disease by strengthening its natural reaction to it, rather than a medicine defeating it without strengthening the body's own resources. It could be said that homeopathy treats the soil, the individual, upon which the disease grows; whereas conventional medicine treats the disease itself without addressing the body's susceptibility or weaknesses.

To suggest that emotional or mental stress during pregnancy could on its own cause a condition as severe as ASD may seem simplistic; however there is research to suggest that stress was passed on from pregnant mothers who were close to the Twin Towers tragedy to their offspring (Yehuda *et al.* 2005).

In auditing his homeopathic practice, the Indian homeopath, Barvalia (2011), divided causations of autism spectrum disorder that he saw into the following categories: physical trauma in children, genetic load, emotional trauma (mother/child), allopathic medication (mother/child), vaccination, preceding infective illness.

One of the challenges that homeopaths face is the difficulty of assessing the disposition of the child when a child is born with or develops symptoms early in life and this can be a reason why family medical history, the pregnancy and mother's state of being during pregnancy can be deciding factors in choosing a homeopathic remedy for very young children. Although every parent knows that each and every child has their own character and habits, it is important for the homeopath to understand this too. Sometimes the isopathic approach may be a necessary part of the homeopathic treatment plan, at other times a nosode may be prescribed and sometimes an individual classical homeopathic prescription.

Philippa Fibert (2012) states that:

> responses to being given homeopathic preparations of these toxins [smoking cigarettes or cannabis during pregnancy, on the contraceptive pill when becoming pregnant, on *Clozapine* when pregnant, working in a launderette when pregnant, multiple courses of antibiotics, MMR vaccination] in ascending potencies were dramatic [in a group of 20 children with a diagnosis of ADHD four of whom had a diagnosis of ASD]. (p.16)

Other homeopaths achieve good results without needing to follow this approach.

RUBRICS THAT THE HOMEOPATH MIGHT CONSIDER

To give a clearer understanding of the range of symptoms which a homeopath will consider in analysing the information gained from the detailed case taking, I have listed below an extensive, but by no means complete, list of symptoms that might be taken into account in the analysis. Each of these rubrics, which is a list of indicated remedies for that symptom collated from homeopathic provings and clinical experience, will guide to selecting the individualised homeopathic prescription.

In conventional medicine there is a limited number of options, such as neuroleptic, antidepressant or stimulant medication; homeopaths have a choice of up to 3000 remedies. However, certain remedies are indicated more often than others in the treatment of any particular disease classification. Not only are the 'autistic' symptoms taken into account, but also a holistic understanding of the patient as a whole, rather than individual parts. This is discussed further in Chapter seven under what the homeopath will need to know. Homeopaths reading this book will find this list of rubrics a useful reference.

Note

As with any system of referencing, rubrics can look confusing at first. Rubrics are written backwards, the keyword being put first. For example 'MIND – ANXIETY – beside oneself from anxiety; being' is read as 'Being beside oneself from anxiety' and 'MIND – ABUSIVE – children – parents; children insulting' as 'children insulting parents' found as a mind symptom in children.

Useful Rubrics for Homeopaths
Treating a Child with Autism

MIND – ABSENTMINDED

MIND – ABSORBED

MIND – ABUSIVE – children – parents; children insulting

MIND – AFFECTIONATE

MIND – ANGER – violent

MIND – ANGUISH – children; in

MIND – ANIMATION – aggravates

MIND – ANSWERING – aversion to answer – sings, talks, but will not answer questions

MIND – ANSWERING – disconnected

MIND – ANSWERING – foolish

MIND – ANSWERING – hastily

MIND – ANSWERING – irrelevantly

MIND – ANSWERING – monosyllables; in

MIND – ANSWERING – reflecting long

MIND – ANSWERING – refusing to answer

MIND – ANSWERING – repeats the question first

MIND – ANSWERING – slowly

MIND – ANSWERING – stupor returns quickly after answering

MIND – ANSWERING – unable to answer

MIND – ANSWERING – unintelligibly

MIND – ANTICS; playing

MIND – ANTISOCIAL

MIND – ANXIETY

MIND – ANXIETY – alone; when

MIND – ANXIETY – anticipation; from

MIND – ANXIETY – bed – driving out of bed

MIND – ANXIETY – beside oneself from anxiety; being

MIND – ANXIETY – children – in

MIND – ANXIETY – company; when in

MIND – ANXIETY – crowd; in a

MIND – ANXIETY – driving from place to place

MIND – ANXIETY – sleep – during

MIND – ANXIETY – time is set; if a

MIND – ANXIETY – waking, on

MIND – APPROACHED by persons; being – aversion to

MIND – ASKING – nothing; for

MIND – AUDACITY

MIND – AUTISM

MIND – AVERSION – family; to members of

MIND – AVERSION – persons – certain, to

MIND – AWKWARD

MIND – AWKWARD – drops things

MIND – BEHAVIOUR PROBLEMS – children; in

MIND – BITING

MIND – BITING – him- or herself

MIND – BITING – people

MIND – BREAKING things

MIND – BUSY

MIND – BUSY – fruitlessly

MIND – CAPRICIOUSNESS

MIND – CARESSED; being – aversion to – children; in

MIND – CARRIED – desire to be carried

MIND – CAUTIOUS

MIND – CHILDISH behaviour

MIND – CHILDISH behaviour

MIND – CLIMBING – desire to

MIND – COMPANY – aversion to

MIND – COMPANY – aversion to – desire for solitude

MIND – COMPANY – aversion to – strangers, aversion to the presence of

MIND – CONCENTRATION – difficult

MIND – CONCENTRATION – difficult – attention, cannot fix

MIND – CONCENTRATION – difficult – studying

MIND – CONCENTRATION – difficult – writing, while

MIND – CONFIDENCE – want of self-confidence

MIND – CONFUSION of mind – dream, as if in a

MIND – CONFUSION of mind – identity, as to his

MIND – CONFUSION of mind – intoxicated – as if

MIND – CONFUSION of mind – mental exertion – from

MIND – CONSCIENTIOUS about trifles

MIND – CONSOLATION – aggravates

MIND – CONSOLATION – ameliorates

MIND – CONTRADICTION – intolerant of contradiction

MIND – CONVERSATION – aversion to

MIND – CRUELTY

MIND – CRUELTY – animals; to

MIND – CUNNING

MIND – CURSING

MIND – DANGER – no sense of danger; has

MIND – DEFIANT

MIND – DELUSIONS – fancy, illusions of

MIND – DESTRUCTIVENESS

MIND – DEVELOPMENT of children – arrested

MIND – DICTATORIAL

MIND – DISCONTENTED

MIND – DISCOURAGED

MIND – DISOBEDIENCE

MIND – DISTURBED; averse to being

MIND – DULLNESS

MIND – DULLNESS – mental exertion, from

MIND – DULLNESS – reading

MIND – DULLNESS – understand; does not – questions addressed to him or her – repetition; only after

MIND – DYSLEXIA

MIND – ECCENTRICITY

MIND – EGOTISM

MIND – ESCAPE, attempts to

MIND – EXCITEMENT – anticipating events, when

MIND – FANCIES – absorbed in

MIND – FEAR – elevators; of

MIND – FEAR – alone, of being

MIND – FEAR – animals; of

MIND – FEAR – dark; of

MIND – FEAR – ghosts; of

MIND – FEAR – noise; of

MIND – FEAR – observed; of her condition being

MIND – FEAR – strangers; of

MIND – FEAR – water, of

MIND – FEARLESS

MIND – FOOLISH behaviour

MIND – FRIGHTENED easily

MIND – GESTURES, makes

MIND – GESTURES, makes – automatic

MIND – GESTURES, makes – fingers – mouth; children put fingers into the

MIND – GESTURES, makes – fingers – picking at fingers

MIND – GESTURES, makes – fingers – playing with the fingers

MIND – GESTURES, makes – hands; involuntary motions of the

MIND – GESTURES, makes – repeating the same actions

MIND – GESTURES, makes – ridiculous or foolish

MIND – GREED, cupidity

MIND – GRIMACES

MIND – GRIMACES – strange faces; makes

MIND – HATRED

MIND – HOMESICKNESS

MIND – HURRY

MIND – IRRESOLUTION

MIND – JEALOUSY

MIND – IDEAS – deficiency of

MIND – IDIOCY [term previously used for mental retardation, which is now referred to as learning difficulties]

MIND – IMPATIENCE

MIND – IMPETUOUS

MIND – IMPULSE; morbid – run; to

MIND – INCONSOLABLE

MIND – INDIFFERENCE

MIND – INDIFFERENCE – everything; to

MIND – INDIFFERENCE – suffering; to

MIND – INDIFFERENCE – surroundings; to the

MIND – INDIFFERENCE – welfare of others; to

MIND – INDUSTRIOUS

MIND – INJURING him- or herself

MIND – INJUSTICE, cannot support – children; in

MIND – INTELLIGENT – narrow field; in a

MIND – KICKING

MIND – KISSING – everyone

MIND – KLEPTOMANIA

MIND – LAMENTING

MIND – LAUGHING – immoderately

MIND – LAUGHING – sardonic

MIND – LAUGHING – serious matters; over

MIND – LAZINESS

MIND – LOOKED AT; to be – cannot bear to be looked at

MIND – MATHEMATICS – inability for – calculating

MIND – MEMORY – weakness of memory – done; for what he or she just has

MIND – MEMORY – weakness of memory – expressing oneself; for

MIND – MEMORY – weakness of memory – heard; for what he or she has

MIND – MEMORY – weakness of memory – mental exertion; for

MIND – MEMORY – weakness of memory – names – own name; his or her

MIND – MEMORY – weakness of memory – read; for what he or she has

MIND – MEMORY – weakness of memory – say; for what he or she is about to

MIND – MISCHIEVOUS

MIND – MISTAKES; making

MIND – MISTAKES; making – calculating; in

MIND – MISTAKES; making – speaking; in

MIND – MISTAKES; making – speaking; in – spelling; in

MIND – MISTAKES; making – speaking; in – words; using wrong

MIND – MOANING

MIND – MONOMANIA

MIND – MOOD – changeable

MIND – MUSIC – ameliorates

MIND – NAKED, wants to be

MIND – NIGHTMARES

MIND – OBSTINATE

MIND – OCCUPATION – ameliorates

MIND – OFFENDED; easily

MIND – PRECOCITY of children

MIND – PULLING – hair – desire to pull someone's hair

MIND – QUARRELSOME

MIND – QUIET disposition

MIND – PERSEVERANCE

MIND – PETULANT

MIND – PLAYING – aversion to play – children; in

MIND – QUEER [eccentric or unusual ideas, opinions or ways of dressing]

MIND – RAGE

MIND – RAGE – strength increased

MIND – RECOGNISING – not recognise; does – relatives; his or her

MIND – REPROACHING oneself

MIND – RESERVED

MIND – RESTLESSNESS – sitting; while

MIND – RETARDATION; mental

MIND – RITUALISTIC BEHAVIOR

MIND – ROCKING – ameliorates

MIND – RUDENESS

MIND – RUNS about

MIND – SCRATCHING with hands

MIND – SELF-CONTROL – loss of self-control

MIND – SELFISHNESS

MIND – SENSES – acute

MIND – SENSITIVE

MIND – SENSITIVE – noise; to

MIND – SHRIEKING

MIND – SLOWNESS

MIND – SMILING – never

MIND – SPACED-OUT feeling

MIND – SPEECH – abrupt

MIND – SPEECH – babbling

MIND – SPEECH – childish

MIND – SPEECH – incoherent

MIND – SPEECH – nonsensical

MIND – SPEECH – prattling

MIND – SPEECH – slow

MIND – SPEECH – unintelligible speech; with

MIND – SPITTING

MIND – SPOKEN TO; being – aversion

MIND – STARING, thoughtless

MIND – STRIKING

MIND – STRIKING – himself – knocking his head against wall and things

MIND – STUPEFACTION

MIND – SUPERSTITIOUS

MIND – SUSPICIOUS

MIND – TACITURN

MIND – TALKING – him or herself; to

MIND – TALKING – slow learning to talk

MIND – TEARING – things in general

MIND – THEORIZING

MIND – THOUGHTS – compelling

MIND – TIMIDITY – bashful

MIND – TIMIDITY – public; about appearing in

MIND – TRIFLES – important; seem

MIND – TOUCHED – aversion to being

MIND – UNCONSCIOUSNESS – conduct; automatic

MIND – UNFEELING

MIND – UNOBSERVING [= inattentive]

MIND – UNSYMPATHETIC

MIND – WANDERING – desire to wander

MIND – WEEPING – causeless

MIND – WILDNESS

MIND – WRITING – indistinctly, writes

MIND – YIELDING disposition

EYE – STARING

STOOL – FROTHY

STOOL – MUCOUS

STOOL – ODOUR – offensive

STOOL – UNDIGESTED

MALE GENITALIA/SEX – MASTURBATION; disposition to – children; in

FEMALE GENITALIA/SEX – MASTURBATION, disposition to – children; in

EXTREMITIES – UNCOORDINATION

EXTREMITIES – WALKING – toes; walking on – must walk on toes

GENERALS – CONVULSIONS

GENERALS – PAINLESSNESS of complaints usually painful

GENERALS – SENSITIVENESS – externally

GENERALS – WALKING – learning to walk – late

CHAPTER THREE

HOMEOPATHY AND ASD AROUND THE WORLD

Overview of clinical results worldwide in the literature with reference to Australia, Brazil, Canada, Europe, India, Japan, Switzerland, the UK and the US.

In this chapter I have assimilated and commented on the work of homeopaths around the world. I have researched published papers from many countries and I have been in conversation with a number of homeopaths worldwide as well. Some homeopaths, like many other people in the health field, are so busy in their clinics helping clients on a daily basis that they don't have time to publish. Some US homeopaths find that as many as 80 per cent of their patients are now on the autism spectrum giving them great insight into this diagnosis in practice. Much of any busy homeopath's practice is built by word of mouth and personal recommendation. Other UK homeopaths received successful treatment of their own children with autism and went on to train in homeopathy themselves, and being well known within the autism community, have built up busy practices themselves.

It can be difficult to use standard research protocols when looking at the use of homeopathy, so the material presented in this chapter might be dismissed as anecdotal in nature, however the personal experience of both practitioners and patients worldwide is too valuable to discount. The issue of research is further addressed in Chapter ten.

AUSTRALIA

In her book, *Challenging Children: Success with Homeopathy* (2007) **Linlee Jordan** looks at ADHD, anger, anxiety, physical problems, poor concentration, sensitivity, tantrums, tics and twitches, and six ASD cases collected from a range of Australian homeopaths. This is a very readable and engaging publication illustrated with children's drawings. It is essentially a book of case histories of people with a variety of diagnoses who have been helped with homeopathy. Linlee has contributed Chapter five of this book 'The Holisitc Approach'.

Fran Sheffield has had a series of articles published in the Australian homeopathic journal, *Similia*, where she talks specifically about three well documented cases of autism in depth, and eight cases in less depth. I have referred to her valuable work throughout the book and especially in Chapter one. She (2008, p.22) states that 'in my practice, distress from noise or odours, and poor gross motor skills are often amongst the first things to improve following an appropriate [homeopathic] remedy'.

BRAZIL

Geórgia Regina Macedo de Menezes Fonseca *et al.* of Brazil (2008) concluded in a pilot study 'Effect of homeopathic medication on the cognitive and motor performance of autistic children' that they found 'positive interference of homeopathic treatment in the cognitive, motor and behavioural performance of autistic patients' and 'even in teenagers, homeopathic treatment positively affected behaviour, with a decrease in aberrant behaviour and better social and familiar integration' (p.70).

CANADA

The Canadian homeopath, **Louis Klein**, presented a case in the German journal *Spectrum of Homeopathy* (2010). He has also looked at specific remedy groups for children with complex developmental and behavioural disturbances and lectures internationally on this subject. Following homeopathic principles he is searching for new remedies that match this pathology in nature. He has lectured on some of his cases where he achieved good results with single remedies in high potencies; but it appears that few of these cases have been published.

EUROPE

A number of successful cases are presented in the German journal *Spectrum of Homeopathy* (Scholten 2010; Schubert 2010; Weiland 2010; Welte and Kuntosch 2010) using the *Lanthanide* remedies in particular. Tinus Smits the founder of CEASE therapy worked with over 300 children before his untimely death. CEASE therapy is discussed in Chapter ten.

INDIA

Dr. M.A. Rajalakshmi, who worked as consultant to a special school in addition to her private practice, shares her findings (2007) of the overall results seen after classical homeopathic treatment as:

- reduction in hyperactivity

- improvement in sitting tolerance/attention span

- improvement in sensory perceptual skills

- better and appropriate expression of emotions

- improvement in both fine motor and gross motor abilities

- improvement in social skills/eye contact

- improvement in speech, language and communication skills

- reduction in anxiety states/temper tantrums

- better sleep patterns.

She concludes that 'internal treatment with Homeopathy that is dynamic in nature possibly helps bring a quick recovery of mild spectrum disorders, and offers a glimmer of hope for even the severe end of the spectrum (e.g. in children who are nonverbal/

low-functioning)'. With a 'possible reduction in effort on the part of the child, the therapist and the parents with improved gains'. She uses the classical homeopathic approach. Progress was assessed using the Autism Treatment Evaluation Checklist (Rimland and Edelson 1999).

Dr Neeraj Gupta in an article entitled 'Homoeopathic medicinal treatment of autism', Gupta *et al.* 2010 concluded that 'our study found significant reduction in behavioural symptoms in Anger/ Biting/Pinching/Hitting) after following homeopathic therapeutic regimen' (p.23). And:

> psychological assessment evaluation observed significant improvement of social and cognitive skills and also showed much reduction of hyperactivity functions and sleep disorders in autistic children. Most remarkable is that autistic children showed constraint and bearable behaviour. Eating and drinking (over eating or no eating) and similarly drinking abnormalities showed significant change. Homoeopathic therapeutic regimen could bring profound control and better coordination in the bowel and bladder especially in cases of nocturnal urination. Also, frequent immunological and allergic reactions which were observed in the autistic children before and during study showed very high rate of protection and very less reactions to allergens. High recovery responses were observed for: gestures, sensory issues (visual, touch and tactile, pain and temperature etc.), audio visual disorders and echolalia. Significant improvement with respect to communication and language skills in the autistic children. (p.25)

Gupta *et al.* (2010, p.24) of the Nehru Homeopathic Medical College and Hospital identified a group of homeopathic remedies found effective in various symptoms of ASD to be: *Belladonna, Bufo, Calc phos, Coffea, Hyoscymus, Kali bromatum, Kali phosphoricum, Phosphorus, Sepia, Silicea, Sulphur, Thuja, Tuberculinum, Veratrum album*. This bears out the effectiveness of the classical approach without needing to use the isopathic CEASE approach.

Dr. Barvalia (2011) of the Spandan Holistic Multidisciplinary Institute treated 123 autistic children and showed that reduction of autistic features and rehabilitation of the child into mainstream society can be achieved through classical homeopathy. He has usefully looked at the affinities of different groups of homeopathic remedies according to the predominant set of ASD symptoms presented. This classification could be very useful in practice especially for the less experienced homeopath. Some of the remedies are discussed in more detail in Chapter nine.

Sensory pattern

Asarum, Borax, Carcinosin, China officinalis, Nux vomica, Opium, Phosphorus, Stramonium, Theridion.

Kinetic state and stereotype

Aurum metalicum, Belladonna, Cina maritima, Tarentula hispanica, Stramonium, Tuberculinum, Medorrhinum, Nux vomica.

Regressive state

Baryta carbonica, Bufo rana, Hyoscymus niger, Zincum metalicum.

Core remedies

Carcinosin, Natrum muriaticum, Medorrhinum, Tuberculinum bovinum.

Auditing 60 cases the first prescriptions were as follows: *Carcinosin, Stramonium, Hyoscymus, Nux vomica, Tarentula, Phosphorus, Tuberculinum* and *Natrum muriaticum.* (p.23)

ISRAEL

Danny Dushan Ron (2013) in Israel is having good results with a Candida-based remedy. He has treated thousands of children with homeopathy at the Israeli Society for Autistic Children and has developed a remedy called '*Candida mix*'. After receiving the remedy he says:

> most patients showed improvements in areas such as: attention-span, ability to concentrate, hyperactivity, sleep disorders and eating disorders [widened variety of foods eaten]... improvements on the physical level with amelioration of abdominal pain, gas, bloating, diarrhoea, chronic constipation and incontinence (both urinary and faecal). (p.14)

He finds the remedy very useful to clear miasmatic obstacles and allows the indicated remedy based on totality of symptoms to work better. He writes in more depth about his work in Chapter four.

JAPAN

The renowned Japanese homeopath, **Dr. Yui** finds that in her experience the complexities of modern diseases need a four-pronged approach. She calls this 'Beyond Hahnemann, the three dimensional method' (Yui and Hamilton 2011, p.26).

1. Remedies for iatrogenic diseases (to remove the ill effects of vaccines and drugs).

2. Remedies supporting organs (to help organs discharge and excrete wastes).

3. Remedies for miasms (to remove tendencies to get diseases).

4. Main remedies (especially *Mercurius* for developmental problems).

In most cases she appears to give three or four different remedies daily. Personally I prefer to give one remedy at a time and to assess its action before prescribing another. However her results documented on video are certainly impressive. Auditing 99 cases of developmental disorder (these may not have been exclusively ASD cases) she found: 60 per cent greatly improved; 21 per cent improved; 8 per cent some changes; 10 per cent became a normal child; 1 per cent new client unknown. (p.26).

She likes to see a clear healing crisis after the remedies are prescribed such as fever or physical discharge or emotional discharge.

SWITZERLAND

Heiner Frei (2005) states in his research project – 'Homeopathic treatment of children with attention deficit hyperactivity disorder' that from a total of 83 patients aged 6–16 with ADHD '70 patients achieved an improvement of 50 per cent or more in their Conners Global Index (CGI). Although these children did not have a diagnosis of ASD, I consider that this piece of research is relevant as symptoms such as 'visual global perception, impulsivity and divided attention' are not uncommon among ASD children. Frei concludes that 'the trial reveals specific effects of homeopathic treatment of ADHD, particularly in the areas of behavioural and cognitive functions. In long-term follow up 74 per cent of all patients did profit of homeopathy without needing any other treatment' (p.2). Successful prescriptions included, in order of frequency: *Calcarea carbonica, Sulphur, Chamomilla, Lycopodium, Silica, Hepar sulphuricum, Nux vomica, China, Ignatia, Mercurius, Capsicum, Causticum, Hyoscymus, Phosphorus, Phosphoric acid, Sepia* and *Staphysagria* (p.13).

UK

Anton van Rhijn (2011) takes a three-pronged approach. First he would change the diet; second provide supplements to aid gut recovery, halt inflammation and correct nutritional status; and third prescribe a homeopathic remedy. Ideally he tries to administer each of these in sequence to assess the effect of each. He discusses two cases in detail in the article and has an excellent and compelling video about his work which can be viewed on Carol Boyce's 'Saving a Lost Generation' (2013) website.

Simon Taffler (personal communication, 20 November 2012, London) who has worked with many autistic children in London and New York says that he likes to see the child communicating as soon as possible, ideally within three to six months of treatment.

He discourages parents from answering questions until the child is given time to respond. He likes to see milestones that indicate first that the patient is listening, followed by eye contact and then yes/no answers followed by simple speech and language development. He likes to see less self-stimming. All of which indicate that the prescription is working. He expects that any tics will stop, but finds concentration problems the hardest to change in his experience. His first goal is to see how the child is communicating with him. Simon writes more about his work in Chapter six.

I have talked informally with other UK homeopaths, many of whom are embracing the CEASE methodology. **Ursula Kraus-Harper** has worked with over a hundred children treated in this way. Like any system it is not always successful, but many experienced homeopaths are finding it a valuable additional tool in treating children with ASD. Generally there is a lack of well collected data as it is a new approach, since it was only launched in 2010. There are many practitioners who have trained in CEASE but still have little practical experience of it. Other homeopaths have been working quietly with a more classical approach.

Philippa Fibert has contributed extensively in Chapter four.

USA

Amy Rothenberg (2010) in her article 'Special kids, special care' writes:

> For children on the autism spectrum homeopathy has much to offer. I have worked with the full range, from kids with Asperger's syndrome to those with profound autism, and almost every child has made some improvement – some subtle, others dramatic. A handful have had such remarkable improvement that their diagnoses were later questioned. I have had previously mute children begin to speak and those who never looked anyone in the eye begin to make eye contact. I have seen many children make gains in their ability to learn and to interact in social settings, and have watched

grateful families begin to enjoy peaceful interaction with their children for the first time. (p.58)

Paul Herscu, Amy's husband, has treated hundreds of children and adults with ASD, which he discusses in his book *Homeopathic Treatment of Autism – Putting the Pieces Together* (2010).

Another American husband and wife team, **Judyth Reichenberg-Ullman and Robert Ullman**, along with **Robert Luepker**, have written extensively about their experience treating children. Their book, *A Drug-Free Approach to Asperger Syndrome and Autism: Homeopathic Care for Exceptional Kids* (2005), refers to 17 well discussed cases and they are very experienced in this field. They follow a classical homeopathy route, searching for a single similimum prescription to address the totality of the child's symptom picture. With their colleague, Robert Luepker (Reichenberg-Ullman, Ullman and Luepker 2005), they write that they have found the following:

> Highly likely to improve with homeopathic treatment: restlessness, mood changes, impulsivity, concentration difficulties, school performance, angry outbursts, oppositional behaviour, socially inappropriate behaviour, most physical complaints, hypersensitivity, confidence and self-esteem issues, awkwardness in interpersonal relationships, social isolation, ability to make friends, obsessive behaviour, inability to participate in team sports. Will probably get better with Homeopathic Treatment: perseveration, eye contact, learning disabilities, pickiness, self-stimulatory behaviour, tics, hyperfocus on special interests, encopresis, bedwetting and echolalia. You may possibly see changes with homeopathic treatment: developmental delays, pedantic speech, lack of empathy and inability to speak. (pp.47–48)

Pierre Fontaine (2012) has defined ASD for the purpose of reversing it as 'spontaneous eye contact, spontaneous speech, spontaneous interaction this is what I call the core' and what he wants to see. He tries to understand the mother's state in choosing his prescription. Although many homeopaths ask about the pregnancy and any problems physically or emotionally during the pregnancy, he specifically asks the mother how she felt at the moment of knowing she was pregnant and how the child's energy felt uniquely different to her own, as a guide to finding the remedy for the child.

Luc de Schepper is another classical homeopath who has worked for many years with children with an ASD diagnosis. He has even developed a 'Homeopathy for Autism' app (2011). He sees the expressions of ASD as linked to the syphilitic miasm (2013). As I understand it he believes that the mother's experience during pregnancy may activate the latent syphilitic miasm. *Mercurius* would be an important remedy as he postulates that the susceptibility to vaccines is linked to the syphilitic miasm.

Looking at his app (2011) he discusses the well-known, to homeopaths at least, polycrest classical remedies such as: *Aluminium, Anacardium orientale, Argentum nitricum, Arsenicum album, Aurum metalicum, Baryta carbonica, Belladonna, Calcarea carbonica, Causticum, Helleborus niger, Lac caninum, Lachesis, Lycopodium clavatum, Mercurius solubilis, Natrum carbonicum, Natrum muriaticum, Nux vomica, Phosphorus, Pulsatilla, Sepia, Silicea, Stramonium, Sulphur, Tarentula,* and *Veratrum album.*

There are many other remedies indicated, that he and other homeopaths would use and this is not a comprehensive list.

In conclusion, there is much work being done by homeopaths around the world, working with children on the autism spectrum. Many of the trials and reports are small scale, but show that positive results are being achieved for these children and their families. The question of research is further addressed in interviews with Carol Boyce and Philippa Fibert and in Chapter ten.

CHAPTER FOUR

CONVERSATIONS WITH HOMEOPATHS

*Interviews with homeopaths about
their experience in the field*

In preparation for this book I have spoken with many homeopaths about their experience of treating children with autism spectrum disorder (ASD). Some have been generous enough to contribute their thoughts in writing for this publication.

CAROL BOYCE MCH CCH RSHOM (NA)

Carol left postgraduate research at King's College London to study at the College of Homeopathy where she graduated in 1985. She was a founder/director of the forerunner of Homeopaths Without Borders UK; she set up teaching and clinical projects from Calcutta to Cairo; took homeopathy to Iraq after the first Gulf war; and taught in medical schools in Cuba. Now a homeopath turned film maker, she produced 'Making a Difference', a film about homeopathy around the world, and is making a documentary series about the potential of homeopathy in conditions like ASD. She is a published author, writing extensively about the politics of medicine, and currently co-founder and head of production at Vitality TV, an online health channel.

I was particularly keen to interview Carol as her documentary film project 'Saving a Lost Generation' is a powerful testament to the power of homeopathy. She has a great overview of what homeopaths are achieving worldwide in the field of ASD, without having a clinic herself, specialising in this area.

What do you see as the limits of nutritional therapy and behaviour modifications?

Nutritional therapy can address deficiencies using supplements and allergens, which produce inflammatory responses, using exclusions diets. Since there is significant bowel involvement in most cases of ASD this makes good sense as an initial intervention. However, as the health of the child improves and the body is better able to assimilate nutrients from the diet, continuing the use of supplements can begin to overload the system and put additional pressure on the excretory system, also often already compromised in ASD.

At a certain point in the healing, the positive effects of approaches like the DAN biomed protocol – where the child may be taking in excess of 30 supplement tablets a day – begin to plateau and then begin to have a negative effect. And that's not even considering the practicality of administering dozens of supplements to small children – or, the often impossible task of adhering to an exclusion diet for a school age child.

As a long term, lifelong solution it is immensely difficult for both the parents and the child, and it seems can only take the child so far. Homeopaths have reported that continuing the bio-med protocol has actually become a barrier to progress at a certain point in some of their homeopathic cases.

ABA therapy is popular and it's easy to understand why. A child that is unresponsive and unable to interact in social situations can learn, via repetition, to adopt certain behaviours that are deemed socially acceptable, allowing the child to become part of the social group. But whatever relief it may afford the child and the wider family in the short term, it doesn't change anything deeper than learned behaviour and in that respect has, in my opinion, serious limitations on how far it can take a child. However, in a family unaware that there are more effective options, it definitely offers the prospect of some improvement, if only in the short term.

What do you see as the potential of homeopathy to reverse autism?

I see homeopathy as having huge, currently untapped potential and I say that based on my experience of speaking to homeopaths about their work and filming interviews with parents of recovered children. Having been involved in homeopathy as a practitioner and a teacher for almost 30 years and in the last several years as a film maker documenting homeopathic work in many parts of the world, I've seen the potential of homeopathy in many conditions, considered difficult or impossible to address from an allopathic standpoint.

The allopathic focus is on the worst aspects of behaviour – the anxiety, the violence, the difficult sleep patterns for example and how to moderate them using powerful medication, which, I would say in most cases, can also compound the problem because of the unwanted side-effects of the drugs themselves. For the homeopath it's a case of looking at the symptoms in each individual case, just as we do with any other condition. Even within the ASD diagnosis there are individualising symptoms, which will lead to the selection of particular homeopathic medicine in a specific potency and dosage.

The cases I have seen are compelling, albeit they are anecdotes – children as old as nine and ten with intractable and severe symptoms of ASD, resolving within days or weeks and moving into mainstream education, without the need for classroom support staff. I have spoken to parents who had tried every conceivable therapy, including powerful allopathic drugs, without improvement and at vast expense – tens of thousands and sometimes hundreds of thousands of dollars/pounds of their own money and without any lasting improvement. Once they see the homeopath the parents describe it as unlocking a door into their child, others describe it as 'getting their child back' – the child they knew before the onset of regressive ASD.

And the changes are lasting and there is continued improvement with minimal ongoing input from the homeopath.

In your overview of what is happening in the homeopathic community worldwide, what do you see people achieving with homeopathy?

In the global homeopathic community practitioners are addressing the challenge of ASD – studies and clinical case reports have come out of places as diverse as India, Brazil, The Netherlands, Australia, the US and the UK. Practitioners report successfully treating hundreds of cases in their own practice. The community is getting on with the work whether it is acknowledged or not – getting good results and publishing their case reports and sharing their experience for the benefit of other homeopaths. There's an urgent need to get this information out – not for any other reason than to let families know that there is an option that they might not yet have considered. The escalating numbers of children affected and the fact that this potential is not being investigated as a matter of urgency by ministries of health is puzzling to say the least.

In your experience what seem to be the most effective strategies that homeopaths use? Can you tell me about specific methodologies that have successfully reversed cases of regressive ASD?

I have met with, spoken to, interviewed and documented homeopaths successfully using a range of methodologies. CEASE therapy, developed by the late Dr. Tinus Smitts of the Netherlands, is gaining ground with a train the trainers programme. Dealing with each layer of potential causation separately makes sense – the environmental stressors, the genetic predisposition, the vaccinations, the underlying constitution and so on.

Others are finding that Dr. Sankaran's sensation method allows practitioners to identify useful homeopathic medicines that they might not otherwise find – while other practitioners are using very straightforward classical prescribing and having excellent results. It's hard to say if any one methodology is more effective than another, they all report recovered children.

One way might be to measure the length of time needed to recover the child, although of course this is fraught with difficulty since every case is different – another measurement might be how well and for how long the treatment holds. At the end of the day it seems the most important thing is that the practitioner should use whatever homeopathic 'tools' they have at their disposal, and utilise them with all their skill.

Do you think that there are specific groups of remedies with affinities for these children?

Like any other condition a homeopath might be called upon to treat, there will be a core group of medicines, which seem to crop up repeatedly – and ASD is no exception. But homeopathy is an individualised system of medicine, and therefore theoretically any medicine could be useful in a specific case of ASD. Having said that I have noticed that medicines like, for example *Stramonium, Natrum Muriaticum, Arsenicum album* and others do come up more often and for some cases can take the child a long way to recovery.

Can you expand on this?

Whether it's useful to know a group of frequently prescribed medicines in any individual case is in question, and might suggest the prescribing is based more on the common symptoms of ASD rather than the individualising symptoms – so there might be temporary or superficial relief but how deep will the resolution be – it's an unknown. Differential diagnosis between a core group of medicines in this kind of situation I think lends itself to the risk of error.

Prescribing on the ASD symptoms would seem to indicate a specific group of medicines, but the differentiation needs to be based on the strange and peculiar individualising signs and symptoms of the case – that will clinch the choice of medicine with the potential to take the child to another level.

What is the most severe case of ASD that you have seen helped by homeopathy?

ASD covers a huge spectrum of symptoms of varying intensity and it depends on how we define severe – in terms of the suffering of the child and/or in terms of the family's ability to cope.

A nine year-old child who wakes screaming every single morning, the slightest deviation of routine results in a minimum of 45 minutes of tantrum including screaming, throwing himself on the floor, banging his head so hard on the floor tiles that he risks serious head injury, walking up to strangers in the park and attacking them violently without warning, parents living in fear that social services will demand he is taken into care. That is very, very hard to manage on a daily basis. The disruption to normal family life is almost impossible to imagine, siblings suffer immensely, one parent must become a full-time carer. That seems severe to me.

A three-year-old, who sleeps 18–20 hours a day, is completely nonverbal, wants to be alone and has no interest in anyone or anything. That is very hard for a parent to deal with emotionally, even though the symptoms are comparatively passive. The family's world shrinks to accommodate a child that can't be in the outside world. Family outings disappear, siblings suffer, strain is put on the marriage.

Seven-year-old twins who are totally nonverbal apart from an unintelligible personal language – can't feed themselves, dress themselves, show or receive affection – lost in a world of spinning tops.

A toddler you can't take to nursery or playgroup because of his violent attacks on other children – by the age of nine this behaviour is much more difficult to manage and in this case, bowel incontinence up to ten times a day compounds the isolation of both the child and the family.

These cases may not be the most dramatic, in fact in the world of ASD they are fairly common, but they illustrate the relentless struggle and challenge day in and day out, year after year – increasingly difficult as the child gets older, bigger and physically stronger. It's not surprising that the rate of divorce is high in ASD families. The effort of making sure other siblings don't miss out on their childhood can have serious emotional and physical consequences for the parents — the sheer exhaustion for one thing — the inability to work — professionals taken out of the workforce to become full-time carers — the whole family suffers in ways it's not always easy to imagine. It begs the question again — why is there no interest in even exploring the experience of these parents — all of the children I've mentioned are now in mainstream education and doing very well — happy, social and integrated into the school community. All these children had previously spent years under other therapies, including allopathic medication. Some therapies had helped, but in a limited way — parents using allopathic drugs had been unable to cope with the severe side-effects and had eventually refused to continue with the medication.

What do homeopaths need to know when treating ASD?

Homeopaths need to be clear about the common symptoms of ASD so that they can individualise the case. They need to be mindful of the sensitivities and triggers when dealing with the child, and acknowledge the amount of stress parents are under — often the direct cause of relationship breakdowns. There is often little outside support for the primary caretakers in an ASD family and even an open acknowledgement of what they go through on a daily basis will count for a lot — both in terms of the homeopathic process as well as the caretaker's emotional health.

Close observation — the perceiving of what needs to be cured, as a homeopath must do in any case. Using adjunct treatment where necessary — dietary changes and possibly supplementation in the short term — can take the pressure off the child, while the homeopathic medicine starts to take effect.

Understanding that these parents (most often the mother) have been on a mission for years, desperately searching for ways to recover their child — they are the experts on ASD. They educate themselves on how to read research articles, many know much more than most medical professionals about ASD and all its ramifications. If there were an advanced degree in ASD most of the parents would pass with flying colours! It's a specific phenomenon – having 'met' and got to know your child in the first years of life, it's devastating to have them disappear before your eyes until they are unreachable, clearly in distress much of the time – often with clear signs of pain and physical anguish – parents will stop at nothing to get that child back – no amount of time, effort and often money, is too much.

What do you see as the causative factors for ASD and how does this relate to homeopathic protocols?

In the documentary work I've done with parents and homeopaths, I've deliberately stayed away from possible causations. I think we have to conclude that causation is multi-factorial and different for each child. The fact that the scientific research is by and large focused on genetic causes does not really tell us very much.

A mitochondrial mutation, which results in fragile mitochondria is interesting, but in terms of solving that child's problem it doesn't help. The homeopath will ask why that mutation occurs in these children. Why is there apparently a startling increase in the number of children with fragile mitochondria?

In the new science of epigenetics many external stressors might be identified that lead to regressive ASD, but then what? How can that shift be addressed with allopathic medicine? In short, I don't believe it can be – only the most difficult symptoms can be moderated and only then with the added burden of serious side-effects.

In individual cases we can suggest certain causations might apply. If the child was developing normally, had multiple vaccines and regressed, and the case resolved using a potentised, isopathic medicine, then it would seem that in that particular case some form of vaccine damage was implicated. Not every child who is vaccinated regresses and not every child with ASD regressed after vaccination but I have heard many, many parents describe that the moment when they noticed their previously healthy child began to regress was within hours or days of a vaccine, and especially following multiple vaccines at one visit. If the jury is still out about the direct relationship between vaccines and ASD (and that issue in itself is a book) I think there is no doubt that the current vaccine schedule is implicated in increasing the susceptibility of children to all kinds of immune system dysfunction, and is likely to be revealed as an identifiable epigenetic stressor.

Partly because the debate about the possible impact of vaccination, for example, is so polarised it would distract from the bigger message, which is that whatever the causation turns out to be, homeopathy has immense potential to help the children themselves – and as a consequence the families, the wider society, the economic impact and so on – the ripples spread a long, long way.

There have been court cases in the US which have found in favour of vaccine damage in cases of autism and an amount of compensation, which might also suggest that there is more acceptance of that particular cause than we might be led to believe in the media for example.

But we do know that not every child who is vaccinated regresses, which then leads us back to the issue of individual susceptibility.

If the child is unable to assimilate nutrients, or excrete toxins from their system – in terms of effective treatment – the homeopath does not need to know which metabolic pathways are involved or why. They need to individualise the case and the homeopathic prescriptions will address whatever those underlying causes are, even if we can't at that point identify them. That's one of the beauties of homeopathy – the child doesn't need to be able to communicate, the underlying causation does not need to be known, and the case can still be resolved because the homeopath needs only the objective signs and the subjective symptoms of the case.

Large bowel involvement is frequently seen in children with ASD – the allopathic prescription of steroids definitely helps with the pain and in turn therefore will also have a positive effect on behaviour and the ability to learn – but in the long term the reason for the inflammation is not resolved and the steroids produce their own problems.

What do you see as the main issues that are preventing the recognition of homeopathy's role in treating ASD?

For many reasons it's difficult for the medical profession to accept that another approach might help in a condition where it has little to offer. The fact that ASD is reaching epidemic proportions compounds this I think. Add to this, the constant mantra in the media, that because homeopathy is currently scientifically implausible it can't possibly work. Careers and reputations are on the line, exploring other avenues of possible solutions risks the ridicule of peers. The current scientific dogma dominated by materialism, which suggests we already know everything there is to know about how the world works, also contributes to the reluctance. I can't help but think that this negative pressure and the fear of peer group criticism, prevents individual doctors from being open to the possibility. It makes no sense that families suffer, relationships break down, children lose a childhood, suffer untold pain, anguish and loneliness because a medical culture is too afraid and closed to even explore a potential solution – even less sense when the solution is safe, gentle, effective and affordable.

Given the current rates of ASD the search for solutions should be at the heart of every health ministry. The economic cost is immense – in the UK the cost of ASD is currently in the order of £26 billion per annum. The vast majority of children with ASD will be unable to live independent lives and the consequent loss of the future workforce impacts society in very fundamental ways. So we need to ask, despite many hundreds of successful cases, what is it that stops the medical profession and the policy makers even looking at the potential of homeopathy while the rate of ASD reaches epidemic proportions?

My own experience getting research off the ground is a case in point.

What kind of research would you like to see to show the effectiveness of treating these children with homeopathy?

There is already a body of research showing the potential of homeopathy – hundreds of case reports that have been analysed, some pilot studies, albeit limited in their scope, have shown significant results.

But we need studies which can test homeopathy in the way that it is meant to be practised. I believe it's both possible and urgent to develop studies that allow both the individualisation of prescriptions and a double blind arm.

My own work with a pilot study has been a long and difficult road without even contemplating the funding required to run the study. Despite the involvement of a respected university department and a very experienced lead investigator (100+ published papers – all in conventional medicine) signed onto the project, we could not get the proposal through the Internal Review Body's ethical board. Not because they were afraid the homeopathic medicines might harm the children, but because there was: 'No evidence in the medical literature showing that homeopathy is useful in the treatment of ASD' and therefore they did not feel comfortable approving a pilot study into the possibility that homeopathy might be useful in the treatment of ASD. The board also wanted the exact prescription and posology for each of the children submitted before approval could be considered, and once the study began the protocols could not be changed. Of course this is like asking a sprinter to race in the Olympic finals wearing wellington boots. The sprinter will finish the race but they won't be able to demonstrate anywhere near their full potential!

It was very difficult to explain the principles of individualised medicine. It would have been easier if we had named a medicine and a potency and dosage that we intended to put on the market at some point in the future. That we wanted to test a system, rather than a marketable product was difficult for the board to fathom and as science contracts rather than expands, it was too much of a 'risk' – not for the children who might have been helped, but for the university and its reputation. It's been an instructive process so far and if I didn't know beforehand how difficult it is to get homeopathic research even onto the starting blocks, I do now.

PHILIPPA FIBERT BED (HONS CANTAB), BSC, MSC, RSHOM

Philippa works as a homeopath in High Wycombe, Northampton and Sheffield in the UK, and specialises in the treatment of behavioural disorders in children. She used to work as a teacher of special needs and then in family education. She has found homeopathy to be the most effective intervention by far for these children and their families. She is currently involved in research into this area, completing an MSc at Goldsmith's University, and is currently a PhD research student at the School of Health and Related Research, University of Sheffield. She is research consultant to the Society of Homeopaths UK.

'Small remedies, big results', about Philippa Fibbert's work, written by Fiona McNeill (originally published in Autism Eye, 2011)

Anita Reynolds' son Connor had always been a bit difficult. He couldn't sit still and concentrate at school and was often irritable with a tendency to focus on just one thing. 'He didn't seem to understand simple instructions, while at the same time being able to understand very complex things,' Reynolds, a child-minder from Northampton, explains. 'When his brother and sister were babies, he wanted to be affectionate but he didn't seem to know how to hold them and gripped them too hard. And he wasn't flexible. We always had to warn him in advance if we were going out somewhere or doing something different.'

Worried that Connor wouldn't cope with the transfer to secondary school, Reynolds finally decided to have him assessed. With a diagnosis of Attention Deficit Hyperactivity Disorder (ADHD) and Asperger's syndrome, she was able, at last, to understand why her son behaved as he did.

However, finding a solution to Connor's problems wasn't so easy. Doctors were keen for him to be put on medication, trying different kinds, some of which made him paranoid and depressed. The school, meanwhile, despite Connor's high IQ, put him in lower sets, exacerbating his boredom and lack of focus.

Reynolds was feeling desperate when, by chance, she came across an advertisement asking for local people to take part in a scientific study looking at the effects of homeopathy on children with ADHD.

Homeopathy, as many of us know by now, is an alternative therapy whereby patients are given minute doses of substances that, it is said, kick-start the body's own healing abilities. Homeopaths prescribe these 'remedies' after exhaustive questioning of a patient's symptoms, habits and emotions and although the treatment is said to be harmless, many people are sceptical about its effectiveness.

Reynolds herself was skeptical, yet, feeling she had nothing to lose, she called Philippa Fibert, the homeopath conducting the research. Connor was accepted onto the study and to his mother's astonishment his symptoms started to improve almost as soon as he started taking homeopathic remedies.

Now, a year later, Connor (now 17) has improved so much that he was recently able to give a presentation at school, something that would have been unthinkable before. He's also started a Saturday job at a local supermarket and the family are able to go on outings together without fear of tantrums and awkward behaviour.

'It's been fantastic!' his mother enthuses. 'It's like we've got the son he always should have been. The homeopathy has helped with everything – his appetite, his growth, his maturity levels. Connor feels so much better in himself, too. Before, it was like his mind was racing so much that he couldn't control himself. Now he can regulate his own moods. I used to worry about him so much,' she continues, 'I thought he might say the wrong things to people when he went out and get into trouble. But now I feel he's going to be OK.'

Working as a special needs teacher and Sure Start adviser, Fibert had always been aware of how little help there was for children with behavioural problems. After having her own children, she decided to retrain as a homeopath and coincidentally, one of her case studies was a nine-year-old boy whose ADHD was so bad that he had tried to kill himself.

'This boy couldn't read, had night terrors and often soiled himself,' Fibert explains, 'But after 18 weeks of homeopathy, most of his severe symptoms had gone. I was absolutely amazed. I thought, "I think I'm onto something here!"'

Now fully qualified, Fibert specialises in treating ADHD. Her current research project has been jointly funded by the Homeopathy Research Institute and Turners Court Youth Trust and because of the overlap between ADHD and autism, some of the children taking part in the study are also on the autism spectrum.

The statistics are being analysed using methods recognised in conventional medicine and so far, she says, the results show significant improvement in patients taking homeopathic remedies.

Even so, Fibert is wary of presenting homeopathy as a miracle cure. 'It can take time to find the right remedy,' she warns. 'This study is very much a process of experimentation and I'm still finding out what works. But after a career trying to help vulnerable children as a teacher and parent educator, I've found this to be the most effective intervention by far.'

Linda Drummer's two children also took part in Fibert's project. Daughter Sally, aged eleven, has ADHD, while son Robin, aged eight, has autism as well as ADHD.

Drummer, also from Northampton, has been gobsmacked by the improvements she has seen in her children's behaviour since taking homeopathic remedies. So much so that she hopes they will soon be able to discontinue their conventional medication.

'It has made a huge difference, not only to their ADHD but to their general health,' she explains. 'It's more than I could ever have hoped for. Within a month we began to see a difference and now, several months into the treatment, my daughter is more organised and can follow instructions. My son's meltdowns have stopped and he's able to explain how he feels using words.'

I interviewed Philippa further about her work, using the same questions that I gave to a number of other homeopaths.

What do you see as the limits of nutritional therapy and behaviour modification?

I see nutritional therapy as improving the 'soil' giving the 'plant' optimum opportunity to grow and flourish. However if the 'plant' was already stunted, even with the best care in the world, it'll never grow into a blooming rose. Nutritional therapy can improve symptoms and allow improved functioning, but this functioning tends to be conditional upon continuing controlled nutrition in my opinion. I have not yet seen a case of autism reversed by nutritional therapy. Maybe Natasha Campbell McBride (Gut and Psychology Syndrome) would disagree with me. However I have had cases where gut dysbiosis was a problematic obstacle to cure and the gut needed improving before homeopathic remedies were effective.

I see behaviour modification as simply helping management of symptoms/difficulties. It can be really helpful, but the problem is still there.

What do you see as the potential of homeopathy to reverse autism?

I see huge potential. However it takes time, dedication on behalf of the parent to see it through, and insight on behalf of the homeopath to correctly perceive the case and remedy reaction. I think it also depends on the aetiology. Some aetiologies are more amenable to homeopathic treatment than others in my opinion.

In your overview of what is happening in the homeopathic community worldwide, what do you see people achieving with homeopathy?

I have heard of notable improvements in overall symptomatology, especially using CEASE methodology, Houston homeopaths, and from Torako Yui in Japan. However in the majority of cases I see homeopathy helping with specific areas such as emotional issues (anxieties, sleep, social problems, etc.); physical (gut difficulties, skin problems); generals (fears, phobias, obsessions).

In your experience what seem to be the most effective strategies that homeopaths use?

No question in my mind that CEASE is really effective where environmental issues play a part, and that tends to be the case with nearly all autistic children. Whether it is that environmental issues exacerbate an already sensitive situation, or are aetiological, I'm not sure, but in many cases improvements in behaviour accompany successful CEASE detoxes.

Can you tell me about specific methodologies that have successfully reversed cases of regressive autism?

CEASE.

Do you think that there are specific groups of remedies with affinities for these children?

I don't think I've seen enough kids on the autism spectrum to comment on this. However with ADHD kids, *Medorrhinum* almost always seems to be the indicated miasm; *Stramonium* has been frequently indicated, especially where there's been trauma (birth or emotional), and surprisingly the *Calcareas*.

Can you expand on this?

Frei in his trial, looked to improve treatment strategies and introduced Boenninghausen's methodology. This increased his prescribing success, and increased how often calc was indicated.

What is the most severe case of autism that you have seen helped by homeopathy?

I haven't seen very severe cases. But I have seen tremendous changes. One child used to have frequent tantrums at any change. The family rarely went out because of him. He had never slept through; he was severely allergic to many things; he didn't go to school because he was so frightened. Over the course of a year all these symptoms disappeared and he is now back at school.

What do homeopaths need to know when treating autistic children?

I think it's important to ensure that they have channels of elimination. I've had problems treating children for example, where they are constipated. Until their bowels are moving properly, CEASE doesn't really work.

What do you see as the causative factors for autism and how does this relate to homeopathic treatment protocols?

CEASE. Environmental toxicity is a huge issue for susceptible children in my opinion. I have one case who is part of a group going through the courts regarding organophosphate poisoning, and this doesn't surprise me. Paul Shattock, research scientist for the autism society, thinks it's a big issue too, and can explain it chemically.

What do you see as the main issues that are preventing the recognition of homeopathy's role in treating ASD?

Lack of comparative research in peer-reviewed journals.

What kind of research would you like to see to show the effectiveness of treating these children with homeopathy?

Pragmatic effectiveness trials (as opposed to placebo controlled efficacy trials) where the totality of the homeopathic intervention is compared to treatment as usual. I would like to build a great big cohort of children with ASD and randomly select different groups to try the different therapies that parents are trying, including homeopathy, to see which are more effective. This is what I hope to do once I've finished my PhD (plug for funding!).

Philippa Fibert has also given me permission to share her PhD research overview: *'Summary of Consecutive case series exploring the effectiveness of homeopathic treatment for children with a diagnosis of ADHD (including 4 with concomitant ASD)'*.

This study asked two questions: is adjunctive treatment by a homeopath more effective than usual treatment after 4 months?; and is homeopathic treatment cumulative (i.e. do children continue to improve)?

For question 1: 20 children with a diagnosis of ADHD received treatment by a homeopath every 6 weeks for 24 weeks and were compared with 10 children with a diagnosis of ADHD who received similar time and attention from the same practitioner. For question 2: treated children continued to receive homeopathic treatment every 6 weeks for one year and their outcomes were compared at baseline, 4 months and 1 year.

Two outcome measurements were used: the Conner's Parent Rating Scale, revised long version (CPRS-R: L) and Measure Your Own Medical Outcome Profile (MYMOP), a patient generated outcome measure.

Results

Question 1: The treated group's results improved over time compared to the non-treated group according to both the outcome measurements used:

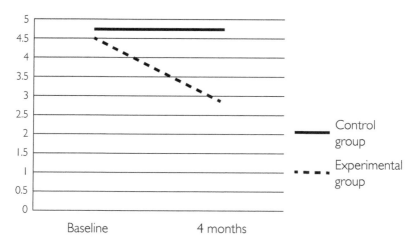

Figure 4.1: Time × treatment for MYMOP scores

[N.B. When collecting MYMOP data from the client they are asked to rate their symptoms on a scale of 0–6, with six being the worst they could be.]

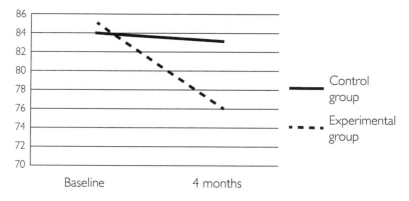

Figure 4.2: Time × treatment for DSM-IV percentiles

Question 2: Treated children's outcomes compared against themselves at baseline, 4 months and one year using T-Tests found incremental improvements at each stage.

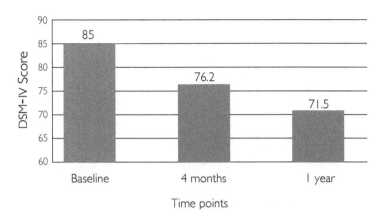

Figure 4.3: Treated children's outcomes compared against themselves at baseline, 4 months and 1 year, using DSM-IV scores

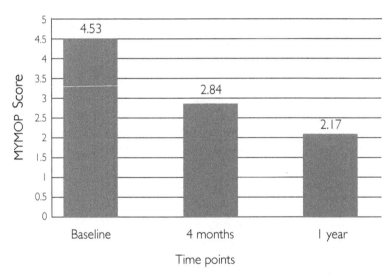

Figure 4.4: Treated children's outcomes compared against themselves at baseline, 4 months and 1 year, using MYMOP scores

Homeopathic treatment

Homeopathic medicines required daily administration initially. It was found that when medicines were stopped, symptoms returned. No potency was found to be more efficacious, and potency was varied according to the sensitivity of the child.

Parents described foetal exposure to the following substances during pregnancy: cannabis and other drugs, alcohol, cigarettes, launderette chemicals and anti-psychotic drugs. Some parents also described changes in their child's behaviour in early childhood, which they attributed to causes such as: emotional trauma, taking asthma drugs, vaccination, antibiotics and certain foods. Specific homeopathic prescriptions were made in consideration of these events in addition to their individualised homeopathic remedies and these specific prescriptions appeared to improve outcomes considerably. Those children whose aetiology was considered to be genetic tended to respond least to treatment.

There were four children whom homeopathy appeared unable to help over the long term and minimal change in scores was recorded after 1 year.

Four children had major improvements in symptomatology after receiving homeopathic potencies of perceived environmental triggers cannabis, antibiotics, salbutamol and clozapine, which had either been taken by the mother while pregnant or by the child, suggesting that homeopathic treatment may be particularly effective where environmental toxicity is suspected as an aetiology. Three of these exceptional responders had a concomitant diagnosis of ASD.

The remaining children experienced moderate improvements The graph below shows score changes in treated children over 1 year (decrease in DSM-IV score indicates improvement). Scores below 65 are considered not to be cause for concern and to fall within the range of normality. Five children fell within the 'normal' range by the end of the year.

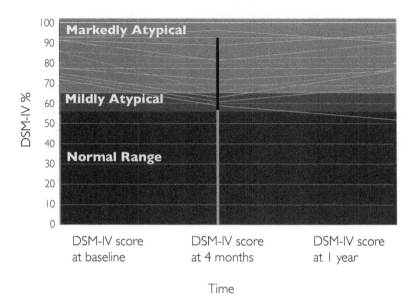

Figure 4.5: Individual DSM-IV scores at three time points

Conclusion

The improvements shown by many of the individuals in the treatment group suggest that homeopathy may be an effective treatment for children with ADHD.

The current study had design limitations concerning the lack of randomisation, the lack of blinding and the lack of objective outcome measurement or collection of outcomes, nevertheless these preliminary results suggest that homeopathy is a useful adjunctive therapy (see Fibert 2014).

DR. M.A. RAJALAKSHMI

Dr. M.A. Rajalakshmi is a registered homeopathic physician from Bangalore, India. She holds a Bachelor's degree in homeopathic medicine and surgery from Bangalore University and a Master's degree in counselling and psychotherapy from Shimoga University, India. She has also gained certificates in music therapy (from Nada School, Chennai), quantitative methods in clinical and public health research (from Harvard University online), and nutrition for health promotion and disease prevention (from University of California at San Francisco online). She has been practising classical homeopathy for over 15 years. She has a particular interest and experience in treating children with autism and neuro-developmental disorders. She has presented research papers on homeopathy and autism in national and international conferences and has also published articles in peer-reviewed journals. She has served as faculty in the holistic therapy unit of a medical college hospital in Bangalore and very briefly as a lecturer in a homeopathic medical college. More recently she ran a homeopathic clinic in the Child Guidance Centre of a rural psychiatric hospital in Calcutta for a year where she also conducted music therapy programmes for residents with chronic mental disorders. She currently lives in Nagpur with her husband who is a consultant neuropsychiatrist.

What do you see as the limits of nutritional therapy and behaviour modification?

Nutrition therapy and behaviour therapy do have their own merits and demerits. If we take the example of the gluten-free casein-free (GFCF) diet where there is total elimination of wheat (gluten) and milk (casein) from the diet, the moment there is an accidental exposure of even a small amount you can see huge aggravation or worsening of the symptoms and you have to start from scratch. This is because instead of stimulating the system to produce the enzymes to digest milk and wheat we are using a temporary solution that may give the system some rest but may not resolve the problem. Instead graded exposure starting with tiny amounts like what has been tried with peanut allergies in children seems to help. This may, like homeopathy, help stimulate the system to heal from within. Of course a proper diet rich in antioxidants and omega-3 fatty acids in natural form has its own benefits. With respect to behaviour therapy, one example that I saw was a behaviour modification strategy of eliminating mouthing in a child with oral sensory issues and the different steps taken to overcome this. The child had an oral sensory issue that was causing the mouthing but that did not seem to be addressed. If the oral sensory issue was treated with homeopathy and then the behaviour modification applied then it would have had more long term and permanent effects. Some stereotypic behaviours like hand-flapping may stem from an internal cause such as tension and I have seen that the behaviours stop after homeopathic treatment even in children where behaviour modification could only help up to a certain extent.

What do you see as the potential of homeopathy to reverse autism?

Homeopathy has immense potential in treating the symptoms of autism. Homeopathic treatment goes to the root of the problem. Since we do not go by just the diagnostic labels and treat the whole child in a holistic manner it is very effective in helping children with this disorder. The other advantage is that it is possible to start treatment at initial stages itself when parents especially mothers start to notice changes in the child. At this stage even if they visit specialists it is not possible to come to a clear cut diagnosis of autism. Of course there have been recent developments in assessment methods where it is possible to predict the probability of developing autism in toddlers (at 18 months). The only option at this stage is starting the child on speech therapy and behaviour therapy. Early intervention with homeopathy would not only help with the symptoms of autism but in some cases might even help prevent children at risk from developing autism in the first place. In my experience of treating children with autism from all over the world in the last 15 years I have seen a number of children who have been integrated into mainstream schools and doing well. Many of them to my knowledge are not on any homeopathic remedy now and they are coping well even after stopping the homeopathic treatment. (I had the opportunity to see a few children after they were integrated into mainstream schools and their mothers said that they continue to progress even without having to take their constitutional homeopathic remedies.)

In your overview of what is happening in the homeopathic community worldwide, what do you see people achieving with homeopathy?

This is the best time for homeopathy and homeopaths. Opportunities for learning and training are more easily available and accessible. There is more awareness about the holistic approach to not only treatment but also to healthy living. People are more inclined to going the natural way and hence a renewed interest in systems of medicine that believe in natural healing such as Ayurveda, naturopathy and homeopathy. Homeopaths have made considerable impact in the treatment of not only autism but many other disorders and diseases. Some major contributions to homeopathy have been achieved by individuals with no institutional backing. If this simple non-invasive method of healing gets the necessary funds and backing of organisations that promote research studies on a larger scale, it will be possible for homeopaths to achieve breakthrough results and find effective solutions for a number of apparently incurable conditions and other complex disorders. There are at least some government-funded research institutions in India that promote research in homeopathy but their publications are not widely distributed and accessible to the general public.

In your experience what seem to be the most effective strategies that homeopaths use?

In my experience both from my personal practice and from what I have seen during my training period, the most effective strategy has been the use of a single remedy at any given point of time: classical homeopathy practice as it is called. Most senior and experienced classical homeopaths use the single remedy, single dose method.

Can you tell me about specific methodologies that have successfully reversed cases of regressive autism?

In my practice what has been most effective is starting with the remedy based on the current symptom picture and doing a review after a month. If there is a change in the symptom picture indicating a change in layer then I change the remedy based on the altered symptom picture and this seems to be most helpful when treating children with autism or other developmental disorders. I also found that daily dosing rather than giving just the single dose has been more effective. Of course I do not universally apply it in every child. I have also used water dosing and alternating remedies when it was required. Using intercurrent remedies such as for example *Bacillinum* or *Medorrhinum* has also been useful in treating specific cases of regressive autism. Homeopathic treatment when used in conjunction with occupational therapy, sensory integration therapy, home behaviour management programmes and other therapies have been found to effectively reverse some of the symptoms of regressive autism.

Do you think that there are specific groups of remedies with affinities for these children?

There are certain groups of remedy. From a broader perspective I have seen remedies from the plant and mineral kingdom have been most effective. Specifically a few of the carbon group of remedies. The other group is a few plant remedies from the *Solanaceae* family.

Can you expand on this?

The remedies I have found most effective in the carbon group are *Calcarea Carbonicum* (calcium carbonate), *Kali Carbonicum* (potassium carbonate) and *Natrum Carbonicum* (sodium carbonate). *Belladonna, Stramonium* and *Hyoscymus* from the *Solanaceae* family have shown good results in children with autism. Apart from that *Lycopodium* and *Silicea* are two other remedies that have worked well. These are not the only remedies and I have used a number of different remedies based on the individual constitutional picture of the child. One observation from my practice I found is that the remedies for late learning to talk like *Natrum Mur.* and for delayed development like *Baryta Carb.* are not that effective when used in children with autism.

What is the most severe case of autism that you have seen helped by homeopathy?

One of the first children I started treating was a child about six years old in the special school where I was a visiting consultant. I would say his was the most severe case of autism that I have seen. This child did not have any eye contact. He would sit in a corner and cry throughout the day. He had a lot of sensory issues and would cry with pain when his socks were removed and put on. His fingertips were also painful. He would not interact or respond when called. He would play with his urine and saliva. In school he would be left alone as the teachers could not do any activity with him. After starting him on homeopathy he first started to respond and be aware of his environment, his peripheral nerve sensitivity came down. He started to interact with the teachers and became a very playful and cheerful child. He would respond very well when spoken to in a musical voice. He started to play music on the drums and his rhythm was perfect. It took about a year of homeopathic treatment for these changes to happen. The dramatic change in this child was the inspiration for me to delve further into finding a homeopathic approach to autism.

What do homeopaths need to know when treating autistic children?

It is very important to know the characteristic features of autism and understand how it is different from mental retardation or other developmental disorders with organic brain damage. If this differentiation is not made, children with autism will be administered remedies that are suited for developmental issues. These remedies will not be effective for children with autism. The homeopath should first get a thorough knowledge about autism before attempting to start treating the child.

What do you see as the causative factors for autism and how does this relate to homeopathic treatment protocols?

There are a number of causative factors currently being postulated for autism namely genetic factors, pre-natal factors such as prescription drugs including thalidomide (thalidomide is still available as a prescription drug for leprosy but is banned for use in pregnant women) and valproic acid taken during pregnancy, viral infections in the mother during pregnancy, poorly developed immune systems in the child, environmental factors such as exposure to toxins both pre-natally and also in infancy. From my point of view after seeing more than about 200 children with autism in my practice I found that the pre-natal stress in the mother during pregnancy does seem to have a significant role to play in the development of autism in the child. This has been corroborated by recent research studies. Vaccines, though there is a controversy, also may play a role from what I have seen and many of the homeopathic remedies for bad effects of vaccination have been useful in children with autism. Many parents have reported sudden changes or regression immediately after the vaccine was administered. I have also noticed that certain events early in the child's life that have a deep emotional impact also led to regression in the child. One parent mentioned that a child who was developing normally up to the age of two years and had developed speech to the extent of reciting prayers in Sanskrit (mantras), completely stopped speaking after there was a family dispute involving his uncle who stopped living with them. He was about three and a half years old when I saw him. In such children remedies that promote emotional healing like *Ignatia* or *Staphysagria* have helped.

Another child was very attached to a tenant neighbour and when he left she became dull and stopped responding, at the same time she also developed a major physical illness with an abscess that worsened her condition when she was about two years old. I saw her at the age of about five years. Once she was treated with the constitutional homeopathic remedy indicated for her she started to improve and she also had a recurrence of her skin condition, which resulted in almost complete reversal of her symptoms of autism. The cure proceeded in accordance with Hering's law. One of my as yet unpublished papers titled 'Theory of Suppression and Miasms as a cause of Autism' talks about the above-mentioned causative factors in detail. There is emotional repression on the one hand and suppression caused by pushing inwards from the physical to the emotional or psychological plane caused by a number of different factors including drugs. The other important factor is environmental exposure to toxins, which could be inhalation of toxins from aerosols in pregnant mothers or a diet with foods that contain toxic additives and preservatives, which has been implicated recently.

What do you see as the main issues that are preventing the recognition of homeopathy's role in treating ASD?

The main issue preventing recognition of homeopathy's role in treating ASD or for that matter any other disorder is the lack of acceptance of the scientific basis of homeopathy despite a number of research studies including basic science research in molecular biology and material science that have helped prove that homeopathic remedies contain quantities of the original substance at a nano level (refer to my editorial review article 'Demystifying homeopathy in the light of nano-science', Rajalakshmi 2012). Another disadvantage is that research studies on the effectiveness of homeopathy for autism are again not accepted because they are qualitative studies and the randomised control trial (RCT) is considered the gold standard. It is not possible to do an RCT with homeopathy as we need to use different remedies for each child. Recently qualitative studies have started to be recognised and that might help in proving the efficacy of homeopathy for autism.

What kind of research would you like to see to show the effectiveness of treating these children with homeopathy?

I would like to see research studies conducted on the changes in the system at a molecular level that happen after the administration of the homeopathic remedy. Research studies that include functional brain mapping to study the areas of the brain that show changes after the homeopathic treatment is started and up to the time that there is most improvement would be very helpful. The other research project that I would like to see implemented is a research project that deals with early intervention strategies with homeopathy for ASD, which will first identify pre-natal factors which could lead to development of autism later in life, and using homeopathy at this stage as a preventive measure or what can be termed homeopathic prophylaxis treatment for children below three years who have been screened using standardised instruments and considered at risk for developing autism.

DANNY DUSHAN RON

Danny is one of the founding staff of Mercaz Adiv (Adiv Center) for Homeopathy and a Healthy Lifestyle. He is a senior lecturer there and instructs interns in homeopathy. He also manages the research unit. Between 1999 and 2001 he specialised in homeopathic paediatric treatment for children on the autism spectrum with various communication impairments (ADD, ADHD, PDD, etc.); he founded a chain of clinics that treat autism at a number of ALUT (the Israeli Society for Autistic Children) branches.

He presents here 'A case study and information about candidemia; homeopathic treatment against candida'.

Abstract

A remedy named *Candida mix*, made from a mixture of fungi and a bacterium, in homeopathic potency, provides improvement in general symptoms in patients with autism.

Background story

My first-born son, Elay, my pride and joy, was born in 1996 after having his head crushed by a violent vacuum extraction during delivery and in spite of my request that he not be vaccinated, without my knowledge or consent, he received a routine vaccination. He was diagnosed with classic autism in 1998. Instead of despairing, I decided to stand up and fight autism. In 1999 I founded a homeopathic volunteer-based clinic for the treatment of autism at Alut. Throughout 1999–2001 I treated hundreds of children in Alut; and up to the present day, I have treated thousands of children and adults ranging from 2–42 years of age, from Israel and other countries.

Candida and autism

A Candida infection is one of the worst symptoms that many children with autism, and children with learning difficulties, suffer from. Candida is a genus of yeast. Many species of candida are normal, harmless flora carried by humans, both internally, mainly in the intestinal tract, and externally, on the skin. However, systemic infections, or overgrowth, can occur and this can have a disastrous effect, especially if the person is already immuno-compromised. Yeasts give off many substances that are toxic to the human host (e.g. zymosan[1], which causes inflammation, and D-arabinitol[2], a

---

1   'Zymosan is a glucan with repeating glucose units connected by β-1, 3-glycosidic linkages. It binds to TLR 2. Zymosan is a ligand found on the surface of fungi, like yeast', http://en.wikipedia.org/wiki/Zymosan, accessed on 20 May 2014.

2   '*Arabitol* or *arabinitol* is a sugar alcohol. It can be formed by the reduction of either arabinose or lyxose. Some organic acid tests check for the presence of D-arabinitol, which may indicate overgrowth of intestinal parasites such as Candida albicans or other yeast/fungus species', http://en.wikipedia.org/wiki/Arabinitol, accessed on 20 May 2014.

form of sugar alcohol) and produce toxins that travel through the bloodstream and affect the brain, nervous system and immune system. The body is no longer able to assimilate the increased levels of toxins and begins to exhibit many distressing symptoms.

Candida is a fungus which, because of the incessant craving for carbohydrates and sugars (the fungus's main form of nourishment) and rejection of other more nutritional foods, causes the child to become malnourished.

In homeopathic terms, the fungus is part of a sub-miasm that belongs to the Cancer Miasm. A direct derivative is the Metabolic-Miasm[3], which is also called the Diabetes Fungus Miasm, and represents the current state of our western world.

From thousands of cases with the same characteristics I deduced the same conclusion – that a key to treating autism may be found in remedies that come from the world of fungi.

The secretion of toxins from the Candida fungus causes hyperactivity, sleep problems and metabolic deficiencies, among other symptoms. Lately we have witnessed a phenomenon in Israel where children on the autism spectrum who ate only bread with chocolate spread began to lose their sight. The main culprit in this case is the fungus that thrives on these sugars; the toxic overload begins to have an effect upon the neurological system causing damage to ocular nerves, and perhaps also contributing to the development of epileptic seizures as well as many other serious conditions. In many cases it is a strong 'obstacle to cure' for well chosen remedies and treatments.

My eldest son also had a stage four Candida infection, which was very severe and was treated with a homeopathic preparation, *Candida Mix*, after which he opened up to all sorts of food, vegetables and fruits, and no longer needed nutritional supplements or special dietary regimes. Eliminate

---

3   The Metabolic Miasm: a new miasm, a sub-miasm from the Syphilitic–Cancer miasm, also called the Diabetes–Fungus miasm, it refers to a state brought on by the diet and lifestyles developed in the western world over the last two to three generations, and now pre-dominant in our collective culture.

the fungal infection and there comes flexibility and working space for the family and the child.

Research and creation of Candida mix

Our research began in 2000 and throughout the course of the research I developed the Candida preparation in collaboration with my friend and colleague Dr. Boaz Ron, a graduate of the Technion – Israel Institute of Technology of Haifa. Professor Israela Berdichevsky from the medical faculty in the Technion, a world-renowned microbiologist and mycologist, assisted and supported us throughout our work.

The homeopathic preparation is produced from various Candida fungus species and from other specific unique bacteria; the remedy is called *Candida Mix*. The preparation clears the fungal infection as well as alleviating the fear mechanism: this is called the 'double restraint' syndrome. The 'fear mechanism' is the result of a physical event in the brain; a part of the brain inside the amygdala[4] is activated initiating a defensive–offensive reaction which causes the child to shut his/her mouth. Literally, the child becomes reluctant to speak, and will often remain silent. The goal of this mechanism is to starve the organism. When the mind and body are in a constant state of fight-or-flight, metabolic crisis occurs and specific neurotransmitters are activated. The body does not seek nourishment, it seeks sugars for maximum calories to feed the muscles and prepare for the assumed crisis; the senses become sharpened and the body is prepared for defence, prepared to survive in a hostile environment.

---

4   Among other brain regions, a deficit in amygdala processing has been suggested to underlie the social impairment, but whether the amygdala is processing fear abnormally in autism is not yet clear, however experiments with animals are confirming anxiety and longer lasting fear memories, which were over-generalised and resistant conditioned fear memories, 'hyperfear', which is harder to extinguish. Fear of this nature may be due to a deficit in the inhibitory system of the amygdala. The researchers have hypothesised an 'aversive world' syndrome that could, even if not a primary cause of the disorder itself, underlie some core symptoms in autism, such as impairments in social interactions and resistance to rehabilitation (Markram *et al.* 2008).

However, this mechanism that is triggered by the Candida fungus is actually a double-edged sword. The delicate balance of the fungus inside the body is lost, and fed by the sugar which it craves, the fungus grows out of control, excretes toxic chemicals and damages the organism, and causes at times irreversible damage. The immune system recognises the fungal infection and attempts to eliminate the toxins from the body. This elimination process may also encompass all of the other chemical toxins and heavy metals that have accumulated in the body due to many circumstances: vaccination, drug use – which can be very high with a special needs child, and air pollution, some of which the child may have taken in during pregnancy, delivery, infancy or early childhood. This places tremendous stress on the immune system, which causes further disturbance or damage to the body.

This system is part of the evolutionary regression that is occurring in the human species, particularly in males. The Candida Mix allows a child to open to a nourishing, diverse diet, to be calmer and sleep better. These are things that are vitally important for the child and his/her family living their day-to-day life, and for the therapists treating the children.

After receiving the Candida mix most patients showed improvements in areas such as: attention span, ability to concentrate, hyperactivity, sleep disorders and eating disorders – having previously had an extremely restricted diet; after the Candida mix they accepted a diet containing a wide variety of foods.

There were also noted improvements on the physical level, with amelioration of abdominal pain, gas, bloating, diarrhoea, chronic constipation and incontinence (both urinary and faecal), all of which are common problems for those with autism.

The main reason for prescribing Candida Mix is to remove an 'obstacle to cure'. Here, for example, is a case study of a very difficult 17-year-old autistic boy.

Case study

Male, 17 years old:

- very violent
- striking himself
- striking others
- biting
- breaking things
- very restless
- sleep disorder.

Medical drugs

The boy receives a regular drug treatment regime including: psychiatric drugs, sedatives and an epilepsy preventative.

Medical history

The patient's mother had been bitten by a stray dog while pregnant with him and had gone to a hospital. There was an argument between the doctors at the hospital regarding the rabies vaccine – was it safe to use on a pregnant woman, or not? Eventually they did vaccinate her and since that day, from a normal pregnancy, it became a very difficult pregnancy with a lot of symptoms on every level: physical, emotional – and mentally she felt like a 'crazy person'.

For we homeopaths, considering the symptoms of her son, it was a clear case of 'mad dog' – it's a case of Lyssinum. I prescribed Lyssinum 200c for the patient. There was immediate improvement after which there was no further change. I understood that I had a case of metabolic miasm – the boy had an eating disorder involving overeating and craving for carbohydrates and sweets; he was overweight, was eating from the floor and was very dirty. We had a Candida test done (faecal test) and discovered that he had a severe Candida infection. I prescribed Candida Mix twice a day for three months, and then we did the test again. The Candida infection had completely cleared and, correspondingly, there was a huge improvement on all levels, of all previous symptoms.

I then prescribed two doses of the Lyssinum 200c, with all symptoms of violence disappearing within two days. The boy started to eat well, sleep well and to show love, sympathy and communication, which he had never before demonstrated – hugs, kisses, smiles and a few new words.

A month later the parents decided, against the advice of doctors, to stop the allopathic drugs.

This case shows how important the Candida Mix is as an anti-miasmatic remedy. The miasm, which included the Candida infection, was the obstacle to cure – it had to be cleared in order to allow the simillimum to work effectively. Today, seven years later, he is still, of course, on the autism spectrum but remains very calm, with no sleep or food disorders, communicative and happy.

This has been our experience of the Candida Mix – it clears the miasmatic obstacles and allows the simillimum to cure the patient.

The Candida Mix

This is composed of several types of yeast and fungi as well as a particular bacterium. We already have *Candida albicans* in the materia medica, but from personal experience, this remedy can help only up to 20 per cent of cases, containing only one species of Candida. However, there are dozens of species of Candida and from tests I have done since 2000, I found the presence of several types of harmful bacteria. The Candida Mix formula is a combination that allows the remedy to deal with all types of Candida with a success rate of 91 per cent.

The potency we have found to be most effective is 6c + 9c + 12c altogether in one bottle. You might call this a homeochord. My experience has been that the 3c factors in potency mixed together gave me the best results on all three levels: physically, emotionally and mentally simultaneously.

Candida infection/Invasive Candidemia

Although best known as a 'thrush' infection in the mouth or genitalia, a Candida infection can happen in almost any part of the body. The infection can also become systemic, spreading to the bloodstream – a condition which is called invasive candidemia. It causes 'flu-like' symptoms including fever and chills, aching muscles, skin rash, head congestion with nasal stuffiness, throbbing headaches, neurological deficits, vision changes or eye infections, abdominal pain, a generalised weakness or fatigue which increases over time and low blood pressure. Weakness of memory and increasing irritability may also be noted. Some sufferers will sometimes experience mental disorders like anxiety or low-grade depression.

Hospital-acquired candidemia is thought to be a major contributor to an estimated 10,000 deaths per year in the US alone[5], and far more than that worldwide. *Candida albicans* is known to be responsible for the majority of these infections. Candidemia is a life threatening infection with high morbidity and mortality, especially among hospital patients who are generally immuno-compromised already. The Candida infection can spread from the bloodstream to other parts of the body (such as the eyes, and the major organs: kidney, liver, brain, heart, etc.) If left untreated the patient's organs may fail and cause death.

Autistic children were reported to have gastrointestinal (GI) problems that are more frequent and more severe than in children from the general population. Although many studies demonstrate that GI symptoms are common in autism, the exact percentage suffering from gastrointestinal problems is not well known, but there is a general consensus that GI problems are common in autism. The observation

---

5   Trofa, Gácser and Nosanchuk (2008).

that antifungal medications improve the behaviour of autistic children encouraged us to investigate their intestinal colonisation with yeasts. The results of our study showed that there was significant relation between the autistic children and heavy growth of *Candida albicans* in stool culture. The high rate of *Candida albicans* intestinal infection in autistic children may be a part of a syndrome related to immune system disorders in these patients.[6]

Once it has been diagnosed, and this may not always be prompt as the symptoms are common to many conditions including 'flu or post-operative recuperative conditions, a Candida infection can be extremely difficult to treat effectively. The cellular structure of fungi is different from that of bacteria, the cell wall of the fungi being rigid, and the cellular membrane resistant to antibiotics. The fungi are also very adaptive and the resistance to drug treatments is increasing so it is not a simple matter of prescribing a course of antifungal medication that will kill the fungi.[7]

A new study by Professor Judith Berman *et al.*[8] at the University of Minnesota and Tel Aviv University shows that *Candida albicans*, previously thought to be a diploid organism (having two sets of chromosomes) which reproduces by dividing without sexual mating, under certain conditions forms haploid cells (having one set of chromosomes and therefore needing a mate to reproduce) capable of sexual reproduction. This important discovery has paved the way for research into new methods of preventing and treating candidiasis and candidemia with more effective higher antifungal drugs.

Thanks

The homeopathic masters Grandgeorge, Vermeulen, Sherr, and of course Klein, all of whom have immense vision

6   Emam, Esmat and Sadek (2012).
7   http://patients.thoracic.org/information-series/en/resources/candidemia.pdf
8   Hickman *et al.* (2013).

and open-mindedness, have given me great inspiration and motivate me to continue my research. I would like to acknowledge the homeopathic laboratory run by the Israeli 'Super Pharm' chain and head pharmacist Yehudit Amara for their help; without them we could not have developed the special preparation.

RESPONSE FROM PROFESSOR ISRAELA BERDICEVSKY

Professor Berediceevsky of the Department of Microbiology, Technion, Faculty of Medicine in Haifa, Isreael writes:

The homeopath and physician Mr. Danny Dushan Ron and Dr. Boaz Ron appealed and asked me to perform and supervise a study on 'Homeopathic treatment against Candida among a diverse population including children and grown ups, and those that were diagnosed on the autism spectrum'. Faeces samples and vaginal swabs were sent to a private microbiological laboratory under the guidance of Dr. Eli Lefler (a senior microbiology PhD and a senior mycologist with huge experience in the field) and Mr. Doron Shefei. The laboratory is located at Elisha hospital in Haifa.

The samples were sent to the laboratory and the results were evaluated quantitatively due to the incidence growth of Candida as follows: negative, weak, middle, massive, massive plus. If the results were positive a homeopathic mixture was prepared individually at the homeopathic pharmacy of Super-Pharm. The individuals were asked to take the mixture for three months. At the end of this period, all the patients had to send again stools for cultivation for the presence of Candida. The patients were asked to keep their regular kind of nutrition.

I would like to remark that I know, personally, Dr. Eli Lefler, and his laboratory, they use qualificated standards, and the results are reliable.

Conclusions

From the table [not reproduced] it can be concluded that 36.1 per cent of the samples that showed massive and massive plus presence of Candida, became negative after the homeopathic treatment, whereas 11 per cent of the samples did not respond at all. A total of 16.7 per cent of the stool samples that showed low concentrations also became negative. More than 91 per cent of the samples showed improvement after treatment.

Summary

From these results it can be concluded that this homeopathic treatment against Candida is highly efficient. This is very important especially among the autistic population, in which Candida is widespread and difficult to treat. I want to emphasise that I know personally some children who have been treated successfully.

CHAPTER FIVE

THE HOLISTIC APPROACH

Staying the long haul

LINLEE JORDAN

THE *NUX VOMICA* STORY

The house I lived in as a trainee nurse was a sprawling Queenslander[1] with lots of rooms and a wonderful conglomeration of verandas. I loved it. Like all the wooden buildings from that era, the stumps underneath created an open area so the house could benefit from the cooling breezes.

Hot summer nights called out for a party to be held under the house. Young interns, nurses and wardsmen all came along. There were varying amounts of alcohol and somehow, maybe with the resilience of youth, we managed to be able to go to work the next day. We thought an occasional hangover didn't interfere with making beds or taking out stitches, nevertheless we were all impressed with our discovery of the 'bear-with-a-sore-head remedy'. We discovered that we could function better at work the day after a party, when we had a dose of *Nux vomica*. That's all we knew about the little white *Nux* pills. We didn't hear the word homeopathy used in conjunction with the pills. It didn't matter. All that mattered was that it worked for most people who tried it. *Nux*

---

1   The 'Queenslander' is a type of wooden house most typical of early twentieth-century Queensland, Australia, characterised by a corrugated-iron roof; highset on timber stumps; verandahs front and/or back, and sometimes the sides. They are now valued as a key element of Queensland heritage and conservation and renovation of Queenslanders is widespread.

was handed out for years until the house sadly got demolished and the other nurses and I moved away.

These days the *Nux vomica* story would be different because we would google it straight away. We would be informed. We would read about the sound and light sensitivity that the remedy helps, we would be happy that it's beneficial for your liver. Then we would try it.

My nursing days are in the background now that I work as a homeopath. Still, after all this time, the best advice about homeopathy is: try it because it works for most people, read about it, ask friends about it but don't get caught up with wondering why it works.

QUESTIONS THAT HOMEOPATHS ASK

After making a choice to try homeopathy, parents are ready to soak up information and it's not always via my efforts to educate them. Just being asked questions in the initial consultation means that they see the importance of taking notice of little things about how their child operates in the world.

Sometimes, the questions may be unacceptable to ask when their child is in the room listening. It might also be hard physically for their child to be in the room for the whole length of the consultation. If the first consult can be just with the parents then consequent appointments can be more child focused.

Some parents might think the questions are a little random, but they all appreciate the genuine interest of the practitioner. Homeopaths have something special sitting in the back of their brain: the knowledge that no observation of a child, however trivial, should be ignored. In fact, the most useful observations include the marvellous quirkiness and differences there are in each individual child.

STRESS DURING PREGNANCY

Questions about a woman's pregnancy sometimes stir up issues that have been silently stewing. Without intending to increase the parents' suffering, if the issues are bought back to life, they help to differentiate between certain remedies. At the same time they illuminate grief, regret, despair and many other feelings the mother has. She certainly might benefit from a well-timed dose of a remedy. Sometimes, we find that the same remedy needed by the mother or father may also benefit the child. Just as important, it is worthwhile for parents to be able to talk about the whole situation and be listened to.

It might seem like an old wives' tale, but Australian research (Ronald, Pennell and Whitehouse 2010) suggests that children born to mothers with high levels of stress during pregnancy are more at risk of developing autism. The research asked about emotions felt by pregnant women during typical stressful life events, such as divorce or moving house. When their children were two years old, mothers completed a child behaviour checklist and it was confirmed that stressful events during pregnancy significantly predicted autistic traits in the young ones.

To further our knowledge on this topic, in our Sydney clinic, we conducted a study (Barron and Jordan 2009), looking at children who had benefited from *Hyoscymus*, which is a remedy given for socialising issues or behavioural problems. Causation factors were studied and there was a high ratio of children, 12 out of 14, who had experienced a traumatic event in utero, during birth or during the post-natal period.

Research suggests maternal stress might act in a way that 'turns on' genes. The stress might be due to life events, physical trauma, alcohol, drugs, cultural or social factors. No matter what the factors are, they change the way the brain works. The stress system defaults to a setting permanently stuck on 'high' or one that is too low. 'However, our genes are not our destiny and with the right strategies, even a behaviour or trait with a genetic foundation can be altered' (Kaiser and Rasminsky 2012, p.19).

The right strategies, in the form of homeopathic remedies, have a beneficial effect on the results of stress. Dr. Farok Master, an educator and homeopathy researcher, is so forthright about this that he titled one of his books: *State of Mind Influencing the Foetus* (Master 2002). Generally, homeopaths are happy to wade into the swamp of emotions knowing it is not a pointless exercise, because our medicines can help people to lift themselves out of the places they get 'stuck' in.

In the clinic, it is the homeopath's job to make people feel comfortable enough to be open about any influences on their child. So my *Nux vomica* nursing party story has been useful because parents hearing about my youthful nursing escapades are more likely to divulge things about which they may feel guilty or ashamed.

An extreme example of the importance of this information was an Attention Deficit Hyperactivity Disorder (ADHD) teenager whose full story is told in the book, *Challenging Children: Success with Homeopathy* (Jordan 2012, p.60). He had been exposed to copious amounts of alcohol in utero and his mother had died from cirrhosis of the liver when he was six. The constitutional remedy he responded to was *Alcoholis*.

THERE MIGHT BE A PROBLEM

Parents who had a pregnancy free from major stress say that they can sometimes see a link between behaviour deterioration and vaccination or antibiotics, but often there is not a defined starting point. It's a gradual realisation that there might be a number of issues with their child due to variable possible causation factors.

Eventually, the child is enrolled in preschool and a teacher starts to make comments about how they have unusual behaviour and the parents can no longer put off getting an assessment. So there is a half-noticed escalation until somebody says 'I think there might be a problem'.

Even if the parents did suspect a problem, when the autism spectrum diagnosis is finally delivered, parents are in shock and go through phases of anger, denial and lots of self-blame. There is also some kind of relief that it is no longer just a doubt. The acceptance phase is when something magic happens and we see the parents emerge as 'google-warriors' who become experts about the individual problems of their child. They discover diet, detox and homeopathy.

THE WORD *SPECTRUM*

The word *spectrum* implies there is a broad range of behaviours between two extremes. The word spectrum also describes the colours of the rainbow, varying from muddy brown at one end right through varying shades of green and blue to the other end with 'show-off' yellow and 'oh-so-clever' orange.

When a child is painting and they haven't got a tube of brown, how do they get that colour? Easy. Add dobs of all the colours onto the tray, and mix them together. It's hard to keep an unsullied colour when the paints have been swirled around and interfered with.

Making use of this homeopathic analogy, at the brown end of the spectrum there are multiple dobs of interfering colours and obstacles to cure slowing things down. At the other end of the spectrum, the brightness of one colour glares so strongly you need eye protection.

Case study: A boy who benefited from *Bufo*

At the 'muddy brown' end of the spectrum was a young boy who was brought to our clinic when he was six years old. During his waking hours, he had to wear a helmet because of the damage he would do to himself from banging his head. Investigations for epilepsy and other conditions found nothing, and a diagnosis of Pervasive Developmental Disorder (PDD) was decided at four years old. His parent's lives were in disarray. They couldn't take him out anywhere and invites to barbecues and social events had stopped long ago.

What were his symptoms and his problems?
If an electrician or a stranger came into the house, he would shriek and run around. Changes to daily routines increased his anxiety and aggression.

- He had severe speech delay.
- He made no eye contact.
- He constantly rubbed himself against furniture.

- He would not drink anything unless there was strong cordial or white sugar added.
- He feared dogs, except for the old floppy dog at home.

What treatment did he receive?

- Speech therapy.
- Respite for the sake of the parents.
- From the paediatrician, a trial of medication to help regulate behaviours and his excessive masturbation. This worsened his behaviour so it was stopped.
- Applied Behaviour Analysis (ABA),[2] with an emphasis on daily living skills; however, when he first presented for homeopathy the parents were having a break from home sessions.
- After commencing homeopathic *Bufo*, dietary changes were easier to implement and the remedy also supported the reintroduction of ABA.

The first response to *Bufo* was that, for days, he produced many foul smelling watery poos and the parents had the washing machine going constantly; his penis was inflamed and his already limited speech was replaced with grunting. It took more than a week for the pooing to stop. When he next appeared back at the clinic, he was not wearing the helmet and the parents had not seen him masturbate for weeks. It was quite a dramatic positive result after quite an aggravation. Through word of mouth, some parents will now come into the clinic wanting an aggravation because they've heard the story of the *Bufo* boy.

---

2   Applied Behaviour Analysis is commonly referred to as 'ABA' and it is a systematic method of supporting and/or altering behaviour. It involves studying behaviour (via observation), analysing the steps involved in producing a behaviour and then teaching or modifying these steps one at a time.

According to Jon Gamble, head banging is a sign of possible vaccination damage (Gamble 2010). Many other children in the clinic have benefited from homeopathic vaccine remedies to remove this obstacle to cure. However, this child's ongoing positive response to the *Bufo* indicated no need for it. After his early improvements, he continued homeopathy for many years and received the same remedy as needed. His anxiety, aggression and speech improved steadily but surely. Against all odds, he was eventually able to enter a mainstream school with a special education class and no longer visits our clinic after moving away.

Case study: A treatment breakthrough for an Asperger's teenager

James is an Asperger's teenager who is far away from the brown end of the spectrum. His favourite colour is a rich green. It is no coincidence, that this green shows in the *Colors in Homeopathy Textbook* (Ulrich Welte 2010) to be the colour associated with the remedy *Rumex*, which a couple of years into his treatment gave a breakthrough in his improvement.

His mother told a story of despair in the first consult and said, 'He has been on a physical–mental see saw.' He was always either physically sick or emotionally having a hard time. James faced challenges at school ever since the kids in the class were old enough to notice that he was quite different to them. He was usually afraid at school and gave no-one a hard time back again, he saved it for home. In his opinion, everyone is against him and at times, he had expressed suicidal ideas.

What were his symptoms and his problems?
- His family history includes ADHD, Asperger's, schizophrenia, borderline personality disorder and a cousin with a label of 'gifted and talented'.

- He has had a cough, on and off, since he was born. Every winter, his mother flies him up to Queensland because the warmth is the only thing that helps him recover.

- He is highly sensitive to many foods, remedies and supplements, and experiences nausea after eating.

- He has a very pale face and deep brown circles under his eyes.

- One of the little quirks he has is to make a loud inhalation before starting a sentence, it interferes with his socialising.

- He is pedantic and often argues the point.

What are the positives?

Together, James and his mum have developed a useful strategy for dealing with current obsessions, which they use in social situations. When he interjects random comments into a conversation she will respectfully say, 'We're not on the topic of colours right now.' If James is upset about the interjection, she just says 'Mmm hmmm' with little eye contact. Next she asks a question, which requires James to engage in the present conversation.

What treatment did he receive?

- Numerous styles of allergy testing in the past.

- Gluten- and dairy-free diet and he had a very limited range of safe foods.

- The first year of homeopathic treatment was repairing his physical state. We would celebrate if a cough would only last ten days.

- Certain reliable remedies used at home were *Apis*, *Chamomilla*, *Ferrum phos* and *Pulsatilla*. They were of great benefit to prevent the need for antibiotics and antihistamines.

- After having a reaction to certain foods to which he was highly sensitive, his mum gave him *Apis* so successfully that he didn't need the usual number of days off from school.

- Hair analysis once a year, at first showing high arsenic and lead, which has responded well to homeopathic chelation.

It was after two years that *Rumex* was tentatively added to his list of remedies. His mother noticed that it improved more than his cough because the pedantic side of him softened. The reason *Rumex* was chosen for him was the peculiar way of covering his head *and* his mouth when he coughs. His mother had taken a video of this in action, otherwise it would not have been seen in the clinic.

Rumex is a homeopathic remedy made from a weed commonly called yellow dock. It has a reputation for the treatment of mucous membrane problems and allergies. Herbalists in the past used it for feeble recuperative powers (Vermeulen 2004). After the *Rumex*, James feels fabulous. Mr Pedantic went on a holiday and left James behind but he had oozing scabs under his bottom lip, which lasted for ten days: a beneficial aggravation. His food range expanded, he had more colour in his face and his physical state vastly improved. It was a long and sometimes rocky road, but now he no longer requires a diagnosis of Asperger's and his mum is going to start studying homeopathy: the ultimate compliment. She has also benefited emotionally and physically from *Rumex*.

WE CALL THEM BAREFOOT HOMEOPATHS

Parents become quite knowledgeable about homeopathy and can sometimes anticipate the direction that the homeopath might take. This is like being partners in the management of their child's healthcare. We call them barefoot homeopaths. They eventually know enough to be able to make some decisions themselves. They might decide to reduce the number of doses when their child is in a phase of all-is-well or to use one of their at-home remedies during a flare up. They also know when to stop the remedy completely and contact the clinic.

It does take a while to get to the stage of barefoot homeopath. Some parents have no desire to learn about remedies as much as that. Perhaps they are exhausted but sometimes they are happy to follow instructions because it feels complicated.

One of the complications is that when parents are still learning about homeopathy, they might feel that giving a lot of doses of a remedy can only be a good thing or at least will do no harm. While it's probably true that it will do no harm, it's also easy to miss the great advantages of doing it right. The best example I've seen of this was one angelic-looking autistic boy whose mum and dad had used *Chamomilla* bought on the internet. The boy had benefited somewhat, so the parents persisted for months using the remedy often. Eventually, the remedy didn't really help anymore. They were discouraged but still they bought him to the clinic and in the first consult discussed the extreme arching of his back when they needed to put him into his car seat or change his nappy and how he would indicate that he wanted a banana or a vegemite sandwich but when they gave it to him, he would hurl it across the room.

It sounded very much like a need for *Chamomilla*. However, careful case taking revealed that he needed a similar remedy called *Cina*. This helped with his disordered bowel and the sickly look about his eyes; it stopped the way he would poke his finger right up into his nose til it would bleed; his restless twitchy sleep improved and also the way he would moan in the afternoon and couldn't be consoled by being carried or soothed.

Even if *Chamomilla* had been a more suitable remedy for him, the long-term care and attention to detail that is required to follow a complex case such as autism is not within the realm of treatment at home.

INFLAMMATION HELPED BY FOUR IMPORTANT REMEDIES

The symptoms of pain, heat, redness, swelling and loss of function are described as inflammation and it does not mean the same thing as infection. It is not yet clear whether brain inflammation actually causes autism but it has certainly been shown to be present. Tests on the brain tissue of eleven patients with autism who had died and spinal fluid from six living children with autism showed activation of immune system responses. Inflammation was found in certain areas of the brain. Autistic children respond disproportionally to stress and things such as certain foods. Then hormones, which are secreted under stress, will stimulate microglia with resulting inflammation (Theoharides, Asadi and Patel 2013).

One of the ways in which a homeopathic first aid kit is useful is when a practitioner is guiding the choice of remedies to help with ongoing inflammatory symptoms. It does not matter where the symptoms come from and they may be due to food, stress, infection, vaccination or environmental toxins. The remedies are chosen individually and are used concurrently with constitutional remedies. From a range of different inflammation remedies, here are four of the most common:

- *Apis*: Puffy, allergic responses where the child feels irritable and restless. Inflammation of cellular tissue, brain, eyelids or lips after exposure to heat, insect bites, shellfish, wheat, etc.

- *Belladonna*: Children who frequently have a fever with a flushed face and shiny skin will benefit by having this remedy instead of antipyretics (anti-fever medicines). Sudden inflammation of ears, conjunctiva of the eyes, throat, meninges or brain.

- *Chamomilla*: Known as a teething remedy although it has a much broader picture. Inflammation of eyes, brain, meninges, ears, glands, gums or intestines.

- *Nux vomica*: Helps nerves (sensitivity to noise, smells, light, touch, pressure of clothes) and also inflammation of the brain, liver or digestive organs. *Nux* might be indicated if there have been a lot of antibiotics, antihistamines, laxatives, etc. (Master 2006).

They are usually not expected to do the deep work of changing the constitution – they are everyday remedies. They do the job of helping the child and family to cope and get on with living.

HOW CAN INFLAMMATION REMEDIES HELP WITH MELTDOWNS?

A meltdown is a common autistic characteristic, not to be confused with a temper tantrum. This is how it goes: Mum cooks an egg for breakfast for her daughter, just the way she always does. She cuts the hardboiled egg in half, just the way she always does. Then, without warning, the little girl starts to shriek about how the egg is not cooked right, she pushes the egg and spoon onto the floor; she slides off the chair onto the floor thrashing around. The girl has forgotten the egg and it goes on for an hour. An innocent egg incident is a trigger for a major meltdown or maybe the mum doesn't notice any trigger.

When a child is in the middle of a meltdown, she can no longer hear anything that an adult is saying. Reasoning doesn't work. She is driven by inflammation or emotions and patterns set in the past. In a meltdown she does not care if those around her are reacting to her behaviour.

When a child is having a tantrum they will look to see if their behaviour is getting a reaction. In a meltdown, the child is burning up inside and the job of the parent is let the heat die down without getting burned in the process. Words can seem to just ignite the problem so talking is not the best option. It's good to act in a way that is the opposite of intimidating. Try to distance yourself psychologically and no matter what comes out of the child's mouth or what they try to do, don't take it to heart. Physically distance yourself if they are being aggressive. As a parenting strategy, don't make eye contact because it can inflame the situation.

Once the behaviour has worn off, the child has had a release, the fire has burned out and a few well-chosen words are important, such as 'I know this is hard for you'. After serious altercations, parents also need to debrief as much as a child does (Kaiser and Rasminsky 2012, p.194).

For kids who have meltdowns, there are a few ways that inflammation remedies are chosen and here are two examples: If it's noticed that the child always has a bright red face when they are in a meltdown, then they may benefit from *Belladonna, Chamomilla* or *Nux vomica*. However, if a pale face is noticed then different remedies are needed.

If the meltdowns occur about twice a week, then a preventive regular dose would be twice a week. If they are every day, then the dose might be given every morning. This anti-inflammation strategy is used as a support for some children.

Case study: Some children receive many different homeopathic remedies

After one month of homeopathy Madhuri was having meltdowns three times a week instead of four times a day, she was eating more and her language was improving. Madhuri was three when she came for treatment and her mum was ready to jump in and do whatever she could. Her cultural background growing up in Calcutta meant that she readily accepts homeopathy.

Madhuri responded quickly but we are continuing her treatment to make sure the changes are sustainable. After three months of treatment Madhuri's mother was saying 'She is like a girl without autism, she will even take a bath'. These days we are helping her anxiety not her autism.

What were her problems?

- Madhuri had severe language delay.
- She repeated things said to her (echolalia[3]).
- She would not speak at all at day care.
- She had a slushy mouth, lots of saliva bubbles.
- She found it difficult to make eye contact, experienced anxiety in company.

---

3   Echolalia is repeating or 'echoing' what another person has said. For example, a toddler who is exhibiting echolalia can quote long segments from a favourite TV show or sing an entire song word for word, but can't ask for a drink when she needs it or answer a question her dad asks her.

- She had chronic pellet-like constipation. She had been on Movicol medication (a laxative) since 12 months old after an episode of faecal impaction when she had a dry, hard stool stuck immovably in the rectum.

- She was very sensitive to textures, there were some parts of the carpet she wouldn't walk on.

- She had a very sweaty head.

- She was sensitive to temperatures, refused to have a bath.

- She was picky with food, smelt her food before eating it.

- She licked metal objects, chewed her hair.

- During pregnancy her mum had high stress levels after the news of unsafe handling of dioxin-contaminated soil close to where she lived.

What does Madhuri love to do?

- She enjoys dancing and loves to sing Hindi songs with her grandmother on Skype.

What treatment did she receive?

- Gluten-/casein-free diet.

- Liquid zinc supplement and magnesium oil rubbed on her skin.

- Homeopathic remedy made from *Movicol* twice a week for two months.

- Speech pathology.

- She has responded well to her constitutional remedy *Mercurius*, or example her sweating has reduced and her sensitivity to textures and different temperatures is no longer evident.

- Her hair analysis showed high mercury and aluminium for which she received homeopathic chelation, supported by the remedies *Berberis* and *Chelidoneum*.

What is her ongoing treatment?

After an excellent recovery like this, we are repeating the *Mercurius* remedy as needed and will continue other future remedies, as needed, over time. Madhuri's mum has begun to give classes to other mothers about gluten-free cooking using some of her traditional meals, but she doesn't have to be fastidious about diet because Madhuri has had no setbacks after occasional forays into a 'normal diet'. (Lansky 2003, p.1)

Forcing children to take a number of supplements and follow a special diet can be a battle. If dietary changes are begun along with a homeopathic remedy, they are easier to maintain, since the remedy itself will be helping to change the child's bowel flora, habits and cravings. This is one of the most wonderful parts of homeopathic treatment. For many children, we anticipate that certain dietary sensitivities will improve along with their other symptoms.

Case Study: In it for the long haul

Thomas first came to the clinic in 1999 when he was seven years old. His diagnosis was Attention Deficit Disorder (ADD) with autistic features. He is now doing an apprenticeship.

What were his symptoms and his problems?

- He would stutter, scowl and have painful-looking facial grimaces when speaking.
- He had no energy and anytime he was in a lying down position like on the couch, he would just go to sleep.
- He had poor comprehension, stared off into space and couldn't remember things.
- He had severe constipation.
- He experienced anxiety and fears of being alone, toilets, dogs, changes to routine, holidays.
- He had excessive saliva.

- He was sensitive to smells, sounds, reprimand, touch.

- He dropped things, had low muscle tone, holding a pencil was difficult.

- He got obsessed by one topic, alternating with no interest in anything.

- He had nosebleeds, only during sleep.

What treatment did he receive?

- Speech pathology, occupational therapy, learning support.

- He has not taken supplements or used a special diet.

- Thomas received the homeopathic remedy *Bovista*. His nose bleeds, facial grimaces, stuttering, sensitivity to smell, constipation, etc. all improved. He responded well to this same remedy in different strengths over many years. At first, due to his sensitive constitution he received 12c twice a day. Later, he responded well to 200c. *Arnica* and other remedies were used as needed, for example after injuries while surfing.

After following Thomas over many years, it is easy to see what homeopathy has done for him. He lost any need for a diagnosis long ago. What we see now is the person who Thomas ultimately is. He's a family orientated young man who is well connected with people.

Our aim in the clinic with any of the children is for them to be themselves and to be happy with who they are, along with their quirky characteristics. We aim to maintain the gains seen early on and achieve a sustained, long-term improvement. This is rarely a smooth improvement, there are usually lots of hiccoughs, with two steps forward and one step back. So long as parents know that this is to be expected, they willingly observe what is going on and report back about it. In anticipation of this we book children in for a check-up every six months once they no longer need active treatment. But after a while, if they *are* doing well, they have other priorities. For example, Thomas sometimes comes once a month for a while to get back on track and then we won't see him for a few years.

COMPLEX CASES

Many children have a convoluted treatment plan, and writing about it and including all of the details is difficult, although we still get positive results. When a child has received just one constitutional remedy like the *Bufo* boy or like Thomas then it is easier to write about. They were probably children who were on the autism spectrum from early in life, which is now less common than children who have regressed later (Ozonoff *et al.* 2008).

Case Study: Alistair, a complex case

Here are a couple of snippets from the complex case of little Alistair, who has been coming to the clinic for three years.

- Following a difficult and traumatic birth, where both Alistair and his mother almost died, his mother grieved the loss of a natural birth and the support of her family who live overseas.

- On a few different occasions, Alistair has responded well to the remedy *Ignatia* 10M (a grief remedy), which helped when he literally refused to eat.

- Throughout his second year, he had recurring bouts of tonsillitis. The ten courses of antibiotics he received is a not uncommon story.

- Alistair would go to the toilet three times a day and he would be straining so loudly that you could hear him down the street but then he would pass a soft stool. His mother was puzzled. *Alum* was a remedy that helped him with this.

- Recently seven-year-old Alistair had a setback after dental surgery, which was done under general anaesthetic because of his sensitivities. Here we see an autistic child needing dental work at a young age, part of the cycle of screaming while resisting toothbrushing and craving sweet foods.

- His hair analysis showed high aluminium and lead levels, for which he received homeopathic chelation supported by the remedies *Chelidoneum* and *Carduus marianus*.

- *Cina, Silica, Bar carb, Psorinum* and *Carcinocinum* all have helped him.

Alistair no longer walks on tiptoes or turns in circles like he had before. His speech is no longer echolalic and there is no more high-pitched screaming or meltdowns, but there are still problems that require ongoing treatment. He remains somewhere close to the spectrum and is doing well.

Case Study: Jeremy, another complex case

Here are some important points from another complex case. Jeremy was born with achondroplasia: the most common kind of dwarfism. His development was progressing well, but before the age of four Jeremy had a regression. He received a diagnosis of autism because he had lost his speech and eye contact, would flap his hands, and screamed at certain noises, etc. According to the parents, he'd also had a problem with his vaccinations especially the chickenpox vaccine.

His treatment included supplements, chiropractic sessions, kinesiology, speech therapy, occupational therapy and he responded to various remedies over time. Most notable were the 'vaccination homeopathic remedies' especially the chicken pox vaccine remedy after which he had a return of eye contact. Another of his major remedies was *Stramonium*, after which his noise sensitivity improved. Jeremy's observant parents noticed that any aggravations always come ten days after a remedy, so potentially deep acting remedies are scheduled at the start of the school holiday period.

The expectation for Jeremy is long-term steady improvement and his parents try not to be disheartened when they notice certain things set him back.

HINTS AND TIPS TO GET THE BEST OUT OF HOMEOPATHY FOR YOUR CHILD

- Have the first consult by yourself to discuss your child's diagnosis, certain behaviours or events in the child's past.

- Give the practitioner a colour photo of your child so they can keep it in their file, it helps when they are working on the case.

- Think carefully about your family medical history, the pregnancy and birth. Write details down and bring a list to the consult.

- After treatment has begun, keep a notebook and write down your observations of your child's behaviour when things happen.

- If your child has a cough, take a video of it on your phone while they are coughing at 2am because when you come in for the consult the cough may be hard to reproduce!

- As much as possible, avoid antibiotics, antipyretics (anti-fever medicine) or anti-anything because sometimes they will cause a setback in your child's progress. If you really can't avoid them, be very aware that a setback is just that and it doesn't mean that homeopathic treatment has stopped working.

- Learn how to use homeopathic remedies at home.

- Introduce dietary changes when you have the support of homeopathy to ease the way.

- Aim for the whole family to go on any special diet together. No cow's milk in the fridge at all!

- Make homeopathy a whole family thing; for example, dad can have a remedy for his eczema, which flares up in times of stress, mum has a remedy for her asthma and siblings have remedies for their jealousy, sugar craving and bedwetting.

SLOW, STEADY IMPROVEMENTS

When we were young nurses, we were on our feet all day, racing from one end of the long ward to the other. After we finished our shift, we sat on the wide veranda of the old Queenslander, chatting and laughing. Sometimes it was too hot to do anything else and talking was therapeutic. We were doing what came naturally to make sense of the events of the day, when we were literally thrown in the deep end of what life dishes out.

In one of the wards, there were many children whose heads were swollen to the size of a basketball with excess cerebrospinal fluid (hydrocephalus). Lots of compassion was required during their bouts of irritability and high-pitched screaming. These days, it makes me think of giving them a good dose of *Apis*. In those days, it was part of our job to turn the little ones over every four hours, because they couldn't turn themselves. Now the techniques of surgically placing shunts to drain the fluid has improved their prospects and the children go on to lead 'normal' lives.

Certain parts of healthcare like that, have advanced greatly since the 1970s, but at the same time certain parts of the health of our children have seen changes for the worse. Since the 1990s, allergy, asthma and autism rates have soared (Kirk 2010, p.57). The search for alternatives in this overmedicated world is becoming urgent and homeopathy offers more than just an alternative.

For the majority of children, homeopathic treatment progresses with slow, steady improvements and a realistic expectation is that enough changes will happen for the child that it will be noticeable. This remains true even for those children who may have dropped nearly all their symptoms but remain hovering somewhere close to the spectrum in the long term.

The *Bufo* boy had an aggravation of his symptoms, followed by improvement, so at first the parents were thinking it's a quick fix, but to consolidate the early impressive changes and translate them into long-term improvement takes time. So the most important hint about getting the best out of homeopathy is to stick with it. It's a process that builds on itself.

Dreams about my nursing days still creep into my night sometimes. Often it's the comfortable old house with the stumps underneath, where homeopathy started for me. In the clinic these days, we have the same kind of chats and laugh like we used to on the veranda all those years ago. 'Debriefing' is what we call it now, and it's much more positive these days, because we can really make a difference for the families who come to the clinic.

CHAPTER SIX

AUTISM OR AUTISMING?

A label or a process?

SIMON TAFFLER

This chapter explains why I advocate homeopathy as a treatment modality for autism. It is a review of my years of practice and the increasing success gained with experience. I have been practising homeopathy since 1985 and I remain constantly challenged by this complex condition, which has certainly provided me with lots of learning opportunities, many disappointments and much joy.

Autism spectrum disorders (ASD) are defined as behavioural disorders characterised by impairments in social communication and social interaction. Those affected have a restricted range of interests with a tendency towards repetitive ritualistic behaviour and atypical reactions to our everyday environment. It is a vast spectrum of behaviours with, for example, varying degrees of eye contact and language development.

Basic ASD is often accompanied by an array of medical conditions and challenges such as seizures, gastrointestinal dysbiosis and sleep disorders. Each and every child or adult with ASD is unique, exhibiting a unique set of symptoms that, one would think, demands tailored care to address specific needs. This is precisely why homeopathy can help.

Homeopaths are specialists in prescribing for the individual. This is exactly what we are trained to do. We don't treat symptoms;

we treat individuals and their unique way of dealing with and responding to their world.

Homeopathy is like opening a window to view a panorama of prescribing possibilities. Accordingly, the profession of homeopathy is peppered with many different styles and prescribing perspectives. Autism is not a standard problem; homeopathy is not a standard product and there are no definitive treatments. Homeopathy may not always produce a miraculous improvement but it can make a significant difference. Indeed in over 25 years of treating patients on the autism spectrum, I have witnessed many positive outcomes.

The prescribing strategy involves drawing on the ASD patient's and their family's experience with a view to solving life, health and wellbeing difficulties. Interventions and supports differ according to the patient's age, array of conditions and level of social and learning skills.

The frequent challenge for the homeopath, is creating and sustaining a relationship with the ASD patient. Forged by experience, homeopaths bring principle and method together with compassion and dedication to the relationship with the family and patient. Of course I can only speak for myself. So let me outline my experience, the principles, the method, and alignment that enabes me to stay dedicated when working with ASD patients who are challenged in life and are frequently challenging to those endeavouring to help, support and guide them.

EXPERIENCE

'It may seem unbelievable, but it's true. My son was cured of an incurable illness.' (Lansky 2003 p.xx)

Those are Amy Lansky's opening words to *Impossible Cure*. Prior to the mid-1990s I had seen a few ASD patients with, frankly, mixed results. My learning was propelled by witnessing Amy's family coping and living with their son Max's autism and by witnessing Max's homeopath, John Melnychuk, prescribe for and support a family in need.

The experience of Max's work changed my prescribing process. I stopped labelling my patients as being on the autism spectrum; rather, they were *autisming* – a process.

Labelling the disease 'autism' and the patient as 'autistic' implies a life-long condition. It is a language and understanding of disease that draws doctors, practitioners, parents and patients into an illness experience overtaken by fear and mechanically minded thinking, one that interprets and labels symptoms and function in terms of 'deficits' and 'disorder'.

Typically parents tell their child's autism story through reports and recorded entries on charts and computers. This is communicated as the official story of the illness. It is as if the allopathic professionals caring for my patients have become the spokespersons for the disease, the patient's stories merely a repetition of the professional's notes and diagnostic criteria, relayed by the parents. An extreme example is of a parent who entered my clinic, sat down and said:

> I've brought you all the reports, photocopied and in date order. That tells you everything.

With ASD patients, many allopathic practitioners have to do something that they are not typically trained to do: tailor the treatment to the individual. They have anatomical, physiological and biochemical knowledge, know standard states of disease and probabilities from evidence-based medicine, yet they are confronted with an ASD human being to whom they must apply their knowledge without their usual tools, because ASD patients are simply not clear-cut.

We are encouraged to follow evidence based pathways, but 'Evidence-based medicine relies…on randomised clinical trials that emphasise efficacy: how an intervention works in a well-defined setting for a specific group of patients with a distinct disease' (Maeseneer *et al.*, 2003, pp.1314–1320).

But ASD patients are a group with an indistinct disease!

It can be so overwhelming and confusing:

> Since the diagnosis I feel I am drowning. Following the tests there has been a tidal wave of reports and information and it's all negative.

> We are so busy. Everything we do revolves around my son's autism. Endless consultants and therapists and we don't feel that we are getting anywhere. I'm confused and I need to find a way out.

Surely if the parents and/or carers are overwhelmed and confused, then the patients must be overwhelmed and confused, which means that the practitioners addressing the ASD issues can become and are often overwhelmed and confused too!

Viewing autism as the process *autisming* enabled me to step out of the drama and put order into my understanding of ASD, into my case taking and into my prescribing process:

> Life-long disorders are recognised, accepted, coped with, and managed. Diseases are detected, prevented, treated, and cured. Diseases are fought, disorders are tolerated. A disorder means out of order. (AutismOne 2013)

Instead of seeing an autistic 'state' or disorder I began to observe the 'process'; to think about autism as a disease process, one that has potential to heal. Or at least shift in that direction.

Homeopaths understand diseases to be a mistunement of the total human condition that can manifest in ways that are seemingly unrelated to each other. To an allopath, a person presenting with compulsive actions, seizures and gastrointestinal symptoms has three problems to treat. To a homeopath there is 'one disease of the whole person' – one problem manifesting in three different expressions simultaneously. This is holism, the treating of disease as a whole-person phenomenon.

Fundamental to the philosophy of homeopathy is the recognition that everyone has an individual, natural, innate healing inclination towards 'wholeness'. Each person's healing process is as unique as a fingerprint.

From this perspective *autisming* is an extreme process caused by the innate self-healing mechanism trying to recover and realign itself.

In my experience, homeopaths who individualise their treatment by studying their patient's way of healing will achieve positive results. This is an attractive proposition that is complicated in practice. Tailoring treatment to ASD individuals is never simple and is invariably challenging for the following reasons:

- There is no definitive treatment, methodology or formula.

- Most cases do not have a clear initiating event.

- Treatment is typically gradual with times of change and plateaus of seeming inaction.

- Managing parental expectations can be difficult as impatience with the treatment process is often the norm; fostering acceptance of the process takes time.

- Treatment usually takes place within a family context of shock, fear, anxiety and desperation.

- Simultaneous use of many forms of intervention, including diets and supplementation, behavioural therapies and language therapies, osteopathy and acupuncture, can confuse if not properly managed.

The goal is a recovery that leaves the person independent and interacting socially without the appearance of new ASD symptoms.

PRINCIPLES

In my opinion, homeopathy is best practised holistically. In other words, cure can only occur by addressing the whole, by prescribing for the complete individual, body, mind, soul and spirit. In practice the homeopathic method involves a specialised 'reading' not only of the presenting symptoms and clinical history, but also of the matrix of interwoven functions and expressions, experienced by the patient and by the family. These might be lifestyle, behaviour patterns, emotional symptoms, physical symptoms, genetic weaknesses and reactions to environmental impressions.

Often, it is small idiosyncrasies, characteristics, discerned habits and mannerisms peculiar to the individual that help differentiate between prescribing possibilities.

This individualised and holistic approach to prescribing respects the mix of entangled processes that characterise ASD patients. It avoids swamping the patient with too much treatment, something that occurs when allopathic prescribers address each problem separately, often creating new symptoms that make the case increasingly complicated.

The challenge for the homeopath is to build an understanding of the patient beyond the obvious, to delve into this very complex condition when there is no such thing as 'normal' and no such thing as a 'normal' family.

Guiding the homeopath are three principles that can simplify the prescribing process: 'causal events', 'obstacles to cure' and 'maintaining causes'.

CAUSAL EVENTS

Causal events are known causes of changed behaviour such as 'my child changed after the vaccination and has been different since'. Twenty years ago, most parents of ASD children believed that vaccination was at the root of their child's condition. Indeed rates of autism increased as the paediatric vaccination protocol grew. There were possible indications that the ever-present mercury adjuvant 'thimerosal' was to blame (Geier and Geier 2006). However, following the removal of thimerosal the prevalence of autism has continued to increase (www.autism.org.uk; Bradford 2013) indicating that multiple factors are probably at work.

While few of my patients have proven vaccine-induced autism, most are highly reactive to an array of substances. I have ASD patients, for example, who were not vaccinated but manifested symptoms following exposure to farming-related chemicals; others were born following probable heavy metal poisoning passing from mother to foetus. Clearly, from conception onwards, there are innumerable possibilities of substances that can compromise immunity and trigger autism. These, together with inherited genetic susceptibility, set children up for an autoimmune response that can manifest in many ways. ASD is multi-faceted, reflecting the fact that many individuals, each with their own disease tendencies and susceptibilities, are reacting to what feels like an assault on their whole system in their own unique way.

OBSTACLES TO CURE

Obstacles to cure are factors that inhibit a curative process and mostly disappear under improved lifestyle or habit, typically an altered dietary regime, drug regime (allopathic) or mental emotional outlook.

Family dynamics, for example, can be an obstacle to cure if they are strongly negative and unsupportive of the homeopathic perspective for treatment. The most common obstacle to cure that is easily rectified is family-wide shock. Following a diagnosis of autism, many parents turn up at my clinic not only shocked, but also fearful and desperate with consequent bonding problems with the ASD child. Parents have said:

> Since the diagnosis my life is at standstill. I can't do anything effectively. I don't know how to look after my kid anymore.

> For months I became obsessed about John's diagnosis, it completely defined me. I read anything I could get my hands about autism, and about people who had success treating it… I'm not focusing on him, only on the diagnosis.

> Our son was slipping away and the best neurology departments on the east coast had no explanation. They offered a bleak future for our son. Our family was tired, frightened and desperate.

> We don't know what's wrong with this child. We don't know what caused it. We have no idea how to fix it.

> He came out of the fit disconnected from the world. Unresponsive with eyes that looked without seeing, ears that heard without listening, with never ending crying, inconsolable. And no help from our doctor…we are praying that you can help.

This state of shock is particularly prevalent in families who realise that they have more than one autistic child or in single-parent families confronted with the balancing act of caring and earning. Homeopathy has an arsenal of great shock remedies for such eventualities.

Deep levels of chronic disease creating a predisposition or susceptibility is the other type of obstacle to cure. Samuel Hahnemann, the founding father of homeopathy, refers to this deeper obstacle to cure as 'miasm' or true chronic disease. The best example that I can think of from my clinic is a family who realised that the common denominator in three generations with ASD symptoms was testosterone imbalance.

MAINTAINING CAUSES

Maintaining causes are unfavourable conditions and circumstances that drain a patient's resources and can antidote the action of remedies. They are factors that create illness by continual exposure to avoidable harmful, often toxic substances. Hahnemann wrote in Aphorism 252: 'Some circumstance is to be found in the regimen or the environment of the patient which must be gotten rid of if the cure is to permanently come to pass' (Hahnemann 1924, translated in O'Reilly 1996, p.224).

The task is to discover what is suppressing natural disease manifestations. Invariably, I look for a product of our modern times like chemicals in food, drink and the environment, air pollution and use of antibiotics and steroids. They all conceivably inhibit the healing process and once isolated, these often unconscious unhealthy practices fade away with improved regimen.

In practice these principles guide the homeopath, who has to gather information from parents and carers unused to divulging the necessary detail, or are bored of retelling their story to different practitioners. The homeopathic diagnosis is always in the detail.

METHOD

The method I use is to follow the patient's lead, typically to follow a child wherever they may take me. I am looking for a way to access their case and build a picture that enables me to prescribe. I am searching for a way to connect. I do this in a number of ways.

Observing

I watch for progress in breathing rhythms, mannerisms, simple sign language, in fact any form of response and communication, gauging against those displayed during the first appointment. I watch for copying and mirroring – skills that indicate development. Newly accomplished copying and mirroring clearly indicates improved understanding, a degree of empathy, improved discrimination and better brain connections. Just learning to copy clapping was a major change for one three-year-old patient, especially when she was also then able to vary the tempo.

In particular I also watch for 'handedness' for different activities. In a world where a majority of the population are right handed, ASD patients are frequently ambidextrous, most are left handed. In a non-ASD person, left handedness normally indicates right hemisphere brain dominance. Yet clinical evidence of left handed ASD individuals strongly suggests right hemisphere brain dysfunction and left hemisphere brain dominance.

The lack of self-awareness, the lack of empathy and inability to identify with others are processes largely associated with right hemisphere resources. So I am watchful for behaviour changes that indicate increased capacity to understand another's thinking, emotions and behaviour. When that happens, I know that new brain connections are being made, that neural pathways are being forged and that positive developments are taking place. For example, one tear-jerking moment occurred when, together with the parents, we realised that their five-year-old son was stamping to say 'yes' with his left foot and 'no' with his right foot.

I encourage parents to observe their ASD child or children and note patterns of behaviour, for example, seizures and vomiting, meltdowns and calmdowns. Recurring patterns of behaviour help identify and often clarify the individual's process, thereby facilitating prescribing. Stopping self-stimming, for example, is often an important milestone.

Listening

I always listen for the different ways that patients express themselves, the vocal ways that they make meaning and survive. Generally ASD children lack empathy and cannot understand social language (resources mediated by the right brain hemisphere) and so lack the ability to convey meaning and feeling through intonation and inflection of the voice. Change in this area indicates great progress.

How language develops is a useful indicator in the homeopathic prescribing process. Most develop speech and language in unusual ways. Some have difficulty combining words into meaningful sentences. They may speak only single words or repeat the same phrase over and over. Many go through a phase where they repeat what they hear verbatim (echolalia).

Most ASD patients learn to use spoken language and all can learn to communicate. Nonverbal or nearly nonverbal children and adults learn to communicate using systems such as pictures, sign language or electronic word processors.

Waiting

Waiting for an answer to a question is an important feature of my clinic. Parents are asked not to answer for their child and certainly not to overwhelm a child with questions, one after another. This generally causes signs of panic reinforcing the notion that ASD children are always oversensitive and overstimulated and have temper tantrums. One teenager after three years of treatment said:

> When I wanted to speak I could not find the words that I needed. I could not answer everything. I got frustrated and just hit out.

I seek some kind of direct communication. A simple response to a question, such as a wave, gives me something to build my relationship on.

From then on a reduction in the time it takes to answer a simple request such as 'Pick up the red car', or question such as 'Which car is red?' is a clear indication of improvement.

I try to avoid failed communications. They usually lead to frustration and challenging behaviours such as screaming or grabbing. Such behaviour usually subsides once the patient has learned to communicate what he or she wants.

Positive dynamics

It seems the misguided belief of many is that the narrower the focus on a particular ASD-related problem, the faster performance will improve. So the teacher, trainer or therapist often directs attention as narrowly as possible, attempting to correct an issue by drawing particular attention to it.

Yet in my experience, over-correcting prevents skill acquisition by focusing solely on what the person does not know, cannot do well or cannot do at all.

Conversely, I've found that highlighting positive behaviours is the best and most effective way to progress ASD children and enable multiple skill acquisition. I encourage parents and carers to highlight positive behaviour and avoid over-correcting and saying 'no' all the time.

ALIGNMENT

My over-riding goal is to develop the right relationship with every patient; one that can be productive and successful. With ASD I need to align myself and the whole family with the healing process of that one person.

I need parents to acknowledge and validate the pace at which their child is progressing, be observant of changes and improvements and frankly have faith in the potential for recovery. Invariably, progress is slow and expectations for change unmet unless I can invite carers and parents to participate and engage in the healing process. Frequently, this causes parents to go on their own journey of self discovery:

> Homeopathy forced me to renegotiate my system of beliefs.

> The more I developed personally, the happier I became and the more he progressed.

> I was led to an understanding that the more I let go of my fears, of my need to battle this autism condition, the more I could accept and trust the process of homeopathic healing.

I align myself to my ASD patients by focusing on the autisming process not the autistic state. Autisming as a process of unusual cerebral organisation, unconventional handedness, unconventional brain function combinations that can lead to hidden positives and unusual talents.

I look to facilitate change from a life of dependency and limited choice to one of independency and choice. I look for milestones that indicate first that the patient is listening, followed by eye contact, and then for yes/no answers followed by simple speech and language development. I look for less stubbornness and obstinacy with cessation of self-stimming. This is a process of increasing connection with the self and with others.

Starting treatment as early as possible improves the chance of a successful recovery. It has been observed that as children with ASD age, they seem to become more distant and it is harder to bring them back. While it may not be possible to 'fully' recover teenagers, it is not impossible to bring significant improvements to older children and adults.

Treating autism can only be a long-term project, taking many months or even many years. The homeopath needs the time to deal with the various facets of the whole and understand the individual well enough to discern the underlying pattern and resonance that lead to a curative remedy or remedies. The patient needs the time to progress to the point where they no longer meet the criteria for a diagnosis of ASD. Often this leads to a diagnosis of attention deficit and hyperactivity disorder (ADHD) or of Asperger's syndrome. Some eventually score within normal ranges on tests for language, adaptive functioning, school placement and personality, but still exhibit mild symptoms on some personality and diagnostic tests.

Sadly, not every child will recover. But I truly believe that homeopathy offers a comprehensive approach and that the right remedy or remedies will bring improvements not possible with other treatments.

> Charlie responded so dramatically to the homeopathy, he no longer needed OT [occupational therapy] or developmental therapy. In fact within six months he was off the diet enjoying what his family and friends were eating.

This chapter presents work in progress. I am constantly learning and thankful to those who provide me with my learning experiences. The challenge of treating ASD patients is substantial but the pay off is huge. Homeopathy has the potential to give a child's life back and save an entire family, and with patience and a strong commitment to the process, allow them to go on to live independent and fulfilling lives.

CHAPTER SEVEN

ASKING QUESTIONS AND MANAGING EXPECTATIONS

Questions to ask the homeopath. Expectations of treatment.
The homeopaths expectations of parents/carers. Working
with non-verbal patients. Frequently Asked Questions.

For many parents or carers the decision to investigate homeopathic treatment is a big step. They may have heard about homeopathy and its potential benefits for children on the autism spectrum on the internet, through an autism charity or from another parent.

In most countries the parents/carers will have to pay for homeopathic treatment as availability of the service is limited. In the UK there are National Health Service (NHS) homeopathic out-patient clinics in London, Bristol, Glasgow and Liverpool, however getting a referral can be a long, drawn out process and availability of appointments may be limited. Many parents/carers choose to pursue private treatment with a suitably qualified professional homeopath; the cost is covered by some insurance companies but not all. However, the cost of homeopathic treatment is not excessive, as appointments are usually four to six weeks apart, rather than weekly and the cost is likely to be less than you might spend on the dentist or vet. In European countries, Australia and New Zealand, homeopathic treatment may be included under national health insurance schemes. In the US, homeopathic treatment is often covered in part by medical insurance.

It is important to check the qualifications and experience of the homeopath you choose; any good homeopath will be happy to talk to you first, before you book an appointment. The main registering bodies for professional homeopathy in the UK are currently the Society of Homeopaths, the Alliance of Registered Homeopaths, the Faculty of Homeopathy and the Homeopathic Medical Association. A list of national and international homeopathic registers and bodies can be found in the appendix.

Make sure that your homeopath's main area of specialisation is homeopathy. Other therapies such as Emotional Freedom Technique (EFT), Flower remedies and Reiki have their place, but to receive good homeopathic treatment you need to make sure that the homeopath has a solid grounding in homeopathic philosophy and therapeutics. Also ask about the length and depth of their training and certification by a registering body. Some homeopaths are also qualified in nutrition and diet, and appropriate supplements are worth exploring both to help with absorption problems and detoxification.

QUESTIONS TO ASK THE HOMEOPATH

What is their experience in working with children,
or indeed adults, on the autism spectrum?

It is important that your homeopath has a good understanding of the different diagnoses and levels of disorder to be able to evaluate changes and be realistic about expectations.

How long will the consultation last?

The homeopath will usually spend one to two hours with you at the initial appointment. He or she will want to spend time speaking to the parents on their own asking questions about medical history, pregnancy and childbirth, developmental stages, any traumas, any similarities with either parent or other siblings. Depending on whether the child is high or low functioning and on their level of communication, the homeopath will want to interact with and observe the child. Some American homeopaths have had great success working with clients long distance by telephone, but this relies on the ability of the parents to give clear information about the child, without the homeopath observing or speaking to the child. Other homeopaths practice by Skype; however in my experience this is not suitable for children, as it is hard to maintain a focused therapeutic space in this context with children.

Should I stop taking my other medications and will homeopathy interfere with any of my current medications?

You should never stop any conventional medication that has been prescribed by a doctor without consulting them first. Homeopathic remedies can be taken alongside, and in complement, to nearly all conventional medication. Homeopathy itself is free from side-effects and can often help with the side-effects of conventional medication.

How do I contact you in an emergency?

Sometimes with a homeopathic prescription, symptoms can flare up but will settle again, however if you are having difficulties you need to know how or who to contact outside office hours. Ask the homeopath about this at your first consultation.

EXPECTATIONS OF TREATMENT

An important part of the homeopath's task is to build a good rapport with your child so that the child will express themselves freely and feel able, as much as they can, to share their inner world.

Homeopaths regard all the symptoms of a patient's condition – mental, emotional and physical – as evidence of a unified effort to resolve an inner disturbance and return to a state of balance. Homeopaths select and prescribe remedies that are known to produce similar symptoms to those of the patient. The remedies themselves are from a variety of sources and are tested on healthy people; there is no animal testing. The results of this testing (called proving) and clinical evidence are recorded in Materia Medica books.

The homeopathic approach to case-taking is very non-judgemental and based on seeking to understand what is unique about each individual client. The child's fascination with a particular computer game may not seem relevant from a conventional medical standpoint. However I recall one particular case of a five-and-a-half-year-old boy who was obsessed with an online dating game, rather than the more usual 'Angry Birds', and composed a very mature love poem the day that his sister broke up with her boyfriend. Taking this sentimentality into account I prescribed a remedy, *Antimonium tartaricum*, after which he started to spend more time playing outside rather than on the computer and forgot all about the dating game. Other important changes also took place in his autism symptoms, such as developing more sensitive communication with others and less repetition of obsessive patterns.

Another child with Asperger's syndrome would take her brother's toys, wrap them up and hide them; she also loved playing with Sellotape, making sticky webs everywhere around the house; this was taken into account in selecting a homeopathic medicine for her. There is no standard treatment protocol for ASD with homeopathy; each person is treated as an individual and their characteristic symptoms and behaviour taken into account in selecting the most appropriate homeopathic remedy for them. How is your child different from other children with a similar diagnosis? It is important for your homeopath to be aware of the common symptoms of the diagnosis and look for what individualises your child.

Parents are often surprised by the kind of questions that a homeopath asks and no-one may have asked those kinds of questions before. Part of their task is to look at how the child's innate potential has gone off course. The child's response to possible causative factors for ASD will be determined by their genetic makeup and the health of parents and grandparents, and each person will have their own inborn susceptibility. If vaccination for example was the cause of autism, why is it that not everyone develops autism?

This is why understanding all of the factors in a child's development and background is important to the homeopath. The more the homeopath knows about the development of your child's symptoms, the easier it is for them to be realistic about their possible prognosis. Based on their understanding and awareness of clinical outcome studies they will be able to assess what type of improvement to expect and how long any improvement might take.

It can be useful to choose a number of symptoms as markers to assess measurement of improvement at subsequent consultations. This may be done more formally through using scales such as MYMOP (Measure Yourself Medical Outcome Profile Paterson) or more informally. One might take for example, a physical problem such as chronic blocked nose, echolalia and self-stimming as symptoms to measure.

THE HOMEOPATH'S EXPECTATIONS OF THE PARENTS/CARERS

Ideally both parents should attend the initial consultation, as each will have their own insights into the child. However, in practice it is sometimes only one parent who attends, sometimes even in opposition to the other parent's intellectual acceptance of homeopathy. It is best to arrange child care for any siblings so that the caregiver and homeopath can give full attention to the patient. Detailed observation of your child is important.

Behaviour in the consultation room should be as unconstrained as possible. The homeopath will set boundaries as to what is and is not acceptable. Some children will try to escape from the consultation room, some may exhibit destructive behaviour, and some will sit on the mother's lap and only answer the homeopath's questions by whispering to the mother, others will indulge in long conversations with the homeopath. The child's drawings or scribbling can be of great use to the homeopath in understanding the child's inner world. Homeopaths prefer it if the parents let the child speak freely without censure, however odd or strange things they say might seem. It will be more beneficial if you commit to a course of treatment; homeopathy is not a quick fix, however desperate you might feel. More will be gained by taking time to build a relationship with the homeopath, giving them the opportunity to offer a well-planned course of treatment to your child. Although parents sometimes start to notice changes in their child within the first few days after taking a homeopathic remedy, to allow for sustained improvement and to progress through a series of appropriately selected remedies will take time. Amy Lansky (2012) said that improvements were noticed in her son in the first few days and months, but treatment lasted over ten years. The initial 80 per cent improvement happened in the initial two years, but the remaining 20 per cent took several more years.

Biomedicine, as discussed in the first chapter of the book, has the potential to suppress symptoms, which can make it harder for the homeopath to gain a clear symptom picture, however if the parents are able to remember what the child was like before commencing biomedical treatment this may not be a problem. Food likes, dislikes and aversions can be a helpful symptom in selecting an individual homeopathic remedy; whereas an allergy or aversion to milk may not be so uncommon, a strong craving for cucumbers might be more unusual. If a food like or dislike is unmodified by notions of what is good or bad for you in terms of food choices, that can be a more valuable symptom to use in selecting a homeopathic remedy than choices based on an intellectual decision. For example someone may choose to be vegetarian as a teenager for moral reasons, whereas another young person may never have liked to eat meat from an early age. This concept is employed in many forms of traditional medicine, for example acupuncture will see the client's likes and dislikes of particular foods as a reflection of the balance of the five elements – earth, air, fire, water and metal within a person's constitutional makeup.

WORKING WITH NONVERBAL PATIENTS

Spero Latchis (2001) reporting on a presentation by Dr. Paul Herscu says:

> With verbal patients, the homeopath may rely heavily on spoken reports of feelings and sensations. With autistic patients, however, pure observation becomes the main tool for case taking. Dr. Herscu strongly stressed the need

to perceive as fully as possible what is taking place in the interview. Following the action/reaction model, the homeopath is the stress and the patient's responses are the reactions or symptoms/signs. Some observations may be quite obvious. Is the patient striking out? Are they verbal? Are they frightened or not? However, it is also important to observe and understand the subtleties of any behaviour you might observe. For example if the child is screaming, why are they screaming? Perhaps they are confused by the newness of the office. The important symptom is then 'confusion' rather than 'screaming'. (p.1)

This raises concerns about relying purely on parental reports to determine the remedy selection, or indeed making home visits rather than having the child come to the surgery. Different homeopaths have tried to deal with the problem of nonverbal patients in a number of ways. Some such as Pierre Fontaine will question the mother to try and understand the child. A question which he uses is 'What was the feeling when you first knew that you were pregnant?' hoping that the mother will have felt the different energy of the child and be able to report on this. Others seem to rely on an inductive intuitive approach. The CEASE approach bypasses this need to find a highly individualised remedy by prescribing on the basis of drug damage (Fontaine 2012). From my experience, if the homeopath can be astute enough, observation of the action/reaction is very effective in working with nonverbal clients. The challenge is then to convert this into useful homeopathic information, without forming suppositions.

I have found it to be helpful when working in a homeopathic teaching environment with a team of other homeopaths, to allocate different roles to the homeopaths or students present in the consulting room. One asking the questions, another observing behaviour and another one observing the homeopath's reactions. It is also useful to listen to one's own inner dialogue. Do they make you feel curious, sympathetic, angry, upset or fearful? If you know yourself well, it is possible to take note of the response a particular patient draws from you and to use this therapeutically. The concepts of transference and counter-transference are recognised in many therapeutic relationships as being valid tools to work with.

FREQUENTLY ASKED QUESTIONS

In May 2013 I conducted an informal question and answer session with parents in the Sussex Autism Group and presented some of the research materials in this area. There may be many more questions that a prospective user of homeopathy may want to ask, but questions asked by this group are helpful to explore with regard to misunderstandings about homeopathic treatment that people may hold. Making the choice to use homeopathy involves a radical rethink for many patients or parents.

What is the idea behind homeopathy? How does it work?

As I have written elsewhere in the book I explain that homeopathy is based on the principle of treating 'like with like'. The homeopath takes an in-depth case history and then matches the characteristics of the remedy to the characteristics of the patient. The prescribed homeopathic remedy will then stimulate the body's dynamic energy system to re-balance itself.

My child has anxiety, is wetting and soiling – would it help?

My personal experience with cases that I have treated is that homeopathy has helped with toileting. The research from India by Gupta *et al.* (2010, p.25) confirms that 'homeopathic therapeutic regimen could bring profound control and better coordination in the bowel and bladder especially in cases of nocturnal urination'. The American homeopaths Judyth Reichenberg-Ullman and Robert Ullman (Reichenerg-Ullman, Ullman and Luepker 2005, p.47) say that in their experience bedwetting is a symptom that sometimes gets better.

How does other medication affect homeopathy?

Other medication can mask the original symptom picture, so homeopaths will often ask how the patient was before they started the other medication. Mixing, and particularly starting, several new treatments at the same time can make it difficult to assess the action of each treatment or medication prescribed. Some homeopaths think that certain substances or medications can 'antidote' or stop the effect of homeopathic remedies. This is something I have rarely seen in my practice, but it can happen very occasionally.

It is not only medication, but also biomedical treatments, supplements and special diets that can hide the full symptom picture which the homeopath needs to be aware of to be able to make the best prescription. It is important not to stop taking any previously prescribed medication when starting on a course of homeopathic treatment. Homeopathy can be used alongside conventional medicines.

Is there any interaction with ADHD drugs?

No. Homeopathy has a long history of being used to help with side-effects or for the after effects of medication that continue after the medication has been stopped. Homeopaths refer to this phenomenon as 'never-been-well-since' (NBWS); this is why a vaccine may be needed in homeopathic form if there is a clearly observed decline in health since a particular immunisation.

Does it take a while to start working?

It can take some time to find the remedy that is most effective. Most patients or their parents/carers observe some changes in the first few days after taking a remedy. In an acute, self-limiting illness, such as an earache, parents can see homeopathy's effectiveness, when for example a child screaming with ear pain experiences immediate relief after one dose of the remedy. This is something observed by parents and homeopaths in thousands of cases. However, more chronic or long-term conditions, which autism spectrum disorder certainly is, will require persistence and commitment on the part of both parents and homeopath. Homeopathy can work amazingly quickly for acute conditions such as stomach upsets, children's complaints, hay fever and so on. However, the longer that you have suffered with a particular problem, the longer it is likely to take to help.

Is it more like an accumulative effect?

This is a complex question to answer. In my experience, once the correct remedy has been prescribed, and this in itself might take some time to find, changes are noticed. However, in the early stages of treatment, there will be periods when symptoms return, partially at least and often of less severity; the remedy may then need to be changed to another, repeated more frequently or in a different potency (homeopathic dilution). It takes time for deep sustained change to be consolidated and for the system to repair. Understanding the homeopathic prognosis and the possibility of change, and case management, require considerable skill on the part of the homeopath. It is not just about finding the best homeopathic remedy to match the patient, but also about knowing how to get the best from that remedy.

What does the treatment involve?

The first stage of treatment is the consultation itself, the homeopath will then analyse the case according to homeopathic principles and prescribe a homeopathic remedy. The homeopath will then need feedback from the parent or carer as to the child's response to the remedy. A series of follow up assessment consultations will be arranged for this. Your homeopath may well offer additional telephone and email support in-between consultations.

The remedies themselves are dispensed in either liquid or tablet/pillule form. Homeopathic remedies come from a very wide range of sources from the animal, plant and mineral kingdoms. Each remedy will have been manufactured according to the homeopathic pharmacopeia. Remedy manufacture involves a process of serial dilution and sucussion known as potentisation. Homeopathic remedies are non-toxic. The process of potentisation produces an ultrahigh dilution of the substance, but no molecules, once the dilution has gone beyond Avogadro's number. The mechanism through which homeopathy works is discussed in greater depth in Chapter ten.

Would you recommend behaviour strategies alongside the remedy?

Of course. Homeopathy however aims at change from within, rather than externally imposed changes. Behaviour therapy might suggest strategies for anger management, whereas after a homeopathic remedy is prescribed, the child's aggressive behaviour may simply no longer be exhibited. Homeopathy is working with the body's own ability to heal itself. It is important to help the child with skills to improve social interaction. It is also recommended for teachers and parents to learn how to interact with the child. Support, both emotionally and practically, for parents is crucial too.

Is it a calming homeopathic remedy you gave to the ten-year-old?

I spoke about the case of a boy with violent tendencies to both himself and others. The selection of the homeopathic remedy is based on an understanding of the whole individual: the core issues and causative factors. Homeopathic remedies are not classified because they are calming, and so on. The individual factors in this particular case which led to the selection of the remedy were his deep jealousy of his brother and his very possessive approach to friends, as well as his violent rages.

Does it nearly always involve tablets?

No it can be liquid doses too. Some children are not good at taking liquids, others are averse to swallowing, so the form of the dose can be adjusted to the individual. The homeopath always seeks to find the most appropriate dosing strategy for each patient, but also needs to take patient compliance into account.

Is there one remedy for all symptoms or one for each?

Homeopathy prescribes on the overall symptom picture rather than on individual symptoms.

Is it similar to vaccination?

Vaccination is treating 'same with same'. It is also using much stronger doses mixed with many other ingredients such as formaldehyde, aluminium, thymersol and others. Homeopathy is treating 'like with like' according to the law of similars rather than the law of the same. Vaccination aims to produce an immune response to one particular disease, or combination of diseases at one time, whereas homeopathy is working on the person as a whole, including their immune system. Isopathy is also treating 'same with same' but without all the other ingredients mixed in and in potentised form. Homeopathy treats each individual case uniquely, whereas immunisation is an undifferentiated treatment of the herd. A homeopathic prescription is based on an existing symptom picture, not on something that does not yet exist or affect the system. Homeopathy is generally observed to raise immunity and resistance, but is not preventative in the sense that immunisation is deemed to be. The controversial topic of 'homeopathic prophylaxis' can be read about widely in other publications and is beyond the scope of this book.

Would you notice a change in the behaviour of the child?

As a homeopath, if I did not see changes in the behaviour of the child I would, in the majority of cases, decide the remedy was not appropriate and seek to find a better suited remedy. There can be cases where the problem is more on a physical level and in those cases physical changes may be noted first.

When research was done around dietary changes and homeopathy; was the research done all together or separately?

In his article outlining a three-stage approach, Anton van Rhijn (2011 pp.97–105) describes following the sequence of treatment below:

1. 'Clean the environment' by changing the diet regime.
2. Provide supplements to aid gut recovery, halt inflammation and correct nutritional status.
3. Homeopathic remedy.

Ideally he tries to administer each of these in sequence to assess the effect of each. He discusses two cases in the article and has a video about his work, which can be viewed on the Saving a Lost Generation website (last accessed 23 September 2013; Boyce 2013).

The article and case studies by Fran Sheffield (2008) explore some of the issues when dietary changes and homeopathy are concurrent, as does the interview with Carol Boyce in Chapter four. CEASE practitioners nearly always recommend a range of dietary changes and a few supplements alongside homeopathic treatment. A clear distinction needs to be made between exclusion type dietary changes such as following a gluten-/casein-free diet or the Feingold diet and the inclusion of a large number of supplements.

Can children be allergic to homeopathic remedies?

No, however, small quantities of lactose, sucrose or alcohol are involved in the manufacture of homeopathic remedies and this might need to be taken into account in the preparation of the remedy for a specific individual and need to be altered to suit their particular sensitivities.

How much would the cost be per month?

This would depend on the country where you obtain homeopathic treatment, how much homeopathy is incorporated into the National

Health Service or covered by your insurance programme, and what the fees are in that particular country. It should be borne in mind that the cost of homeopathy is largely due to the cost of the lengthy individualised consultations and case management, rather than the homeopathic remedies themselves.

Why is homeopathy better than conventional treatment?

One of the great advantages of homeopathy is that treatment is without side-effects. Many parents complain of and are unhappy with the side-effects of prescribed conventional drugs. It is generally acknowledged that conventional medicine offers no cure for the underlying symptoms of autism and that behavioural or nutritional approaches are only able to manage or mitigate symptoms. As this book has shown, homeopathy has at times taken children to a point where they are no longer classified as on the autism spectrum. At other times it may mitigate many troublesome emotional and physical symptoms and all of this without side-effects.

CHAPTER EIGHT

WORKING WITH OTHERS

How homeopaths work with parents, teachers, other healthcare professionals and autism charities.

WORKING WITH PARENTS

Throughout this book I have tried to emphasise that visiting a homeopath and starting the 'homeopathic journey' is very much a collaborative relationship between parents and their chosen practitioner.

Homeopathic case taking involves both the homeopath obtaining the information that he or she needs to make an appropriate homeopathic prescription and the patient or parent being encouraged to share symptoms in the depth required for a homeopathic prescription. As discussed elsewhere in the book, this will involve asking about many areas that can seem unrelated to the problem presented. The homeopath wants to understand what lies behind the 'autistic label' and/or other diagnostic labels. Who is the person behind the label and how do they individually experience their symptoms?

In-depth feedback at subsequent follow ups from the parent or carer and the patient is crucial to enable the homeopath to assess the effect of the homeopathic remedy prescribed. It is not just a case of coming back for more medicine or following the doctor's advice.

In my experience, patients will often phone up or email me after the first consultation and tell me something that they forgot to mention. The homeopath has to be on the alert at all times, the patient may say something crucial just as they leave the room thinking that the consultation is over. This is often referred to as the 'door knob symptom' by homeopaths.

WORKING WITH TEACHERS AND OTHER HEALTHCARE PROFESSIONALS

It is always useful to have not only the parents/carers, and indeed the child's, own assessment of their response to treatment, but also the view of any professionals involved in working with the child. Frei *et al.* (2006) specifically refer to, and make use of 'Teachers' Rating' in their published research paper, 'Treatment of hyperactive children: increased efficiency through modifications of homeopathic diagnostic procedure'. Unfortunately in practice, it is rare that the homeopath receives direct feedback from teachers, speech therapists or other professionals involved in the child's care.

Anecdotally many parents will report, second-hand, that a change in their child's behaviour or concentration has been observed by teachers at school. Or a child psychologist will say 'carry on doing what you are doing, it seems to be working'.

A useful way forward in attempting to work alongside, and to receive feedback from, teachers and other healthcare professionals may be the use of autism questionnaires by homeopaths. The *Autism Treatment Evaluation Check-list* (Rimland and Edelson 1999) is a one-page form that is copyright-free, unlike many other tests. It is specifically designed to be completed by parents, teachers or carers. It consists of four subtests, in the areas of:

1. Speech/language communication (14 items).

2. Sociability (20 items).

3. Sensory/cognitive awareness (18 items).

4. Health/physical/behaviour (25 items).

Other scales that have been used to assess children with autism spectrum disorder (ASD) include: The Childhood Autism Rating Scale (CARS), the Gilliam Autism Rating Scale (GARS) and the Autism Behaviour Checklist (ABC). These assessment tools, which are used in the diagnosis and measurement of autism, may vary in their frequency of use or acceptance from country to country. Determination of Social Quotient (SQ) by Vineland Social Maturity Scale (VSMS) and Psychoeducational Profile Revised PEP-R have also been used by some homeopaths to evaluate the results of homeopathic treatment. The Conners Global Index (CGI) is used more for the assessment of attention deficit hyperactivity disorder (ADHD).

A questionnaire can be a useful way to assess improvement over time; although it may not always be considered a valid research tool, it is a way for both parents and practitioners to keep track of improvements over time. Ideally a questionnaire could also be completed by teachers and other professionals involved with the child to monitor progress. Scoring can be either on a positive or negative scale. The Centre for Academic Primary Care (2013) offers advice on using the Measure Yourself Medical Outcome Profile (MYMOP). This tool, for example, uses a scale of six for the worst a symptom can be and zero for no symptom experienced by the patient. Other scales may use percentage scores to gauge the severity of a symptom, some patients find this easier to relate to, i.e. the symptom is 70 per cent better, or it was a ten and now is only a three. Different patients and practitioners will have their own preferences as to the assessment tool that they prefer to work with.

WORKING WITH AUTISM CHARITIES

The autism charities such as the Autism Research Institute (ARI) and their project Defeat Autism Now (DAN) and Research Autism provide an enormous amount of information for parents and carers. They have tried to evaluate the effectiveness of different approaches that are used by parents of children on the autism spectrum. They seem to have used a mix of patient/carer evaluation and an evidence-based approach. Homeopathy is not well represented or understood on the websites of many autism charities.

However, generationrescue.org and autismone.org have invited speakers on homeopathy to present at their conferences. Additionally, autismone.org has many podcasts in which homeopaths are interviewed about their work and approach to working with ASD children. Carol Boyce has worked in the past with Generation Rescue to provide a database of homeopaths involved in treating autism.

The American homeopath Pierre Fontaine has spoken at the AutismOne Conference in May 2011 and 2012 and at the third Annual Autism Around the World Conference in Dubai 2011.

A video is available on his website (Fontaine 2012). Fontaine's invitation to speak at the Dubai conference highlights the esteem in which homeopathy is held in different cultures. There is still a strong tradition of more natural approaches to health in many Asian and Arabic nations and indeed homeopathy continues to grow in the developing economies world. Homeopathy is at least partially integrated into more mainstream healthcare in India, and the contribution of homeopaths is more recognised than might seem the case in the UK, Australia and the USA.

The Indian homeopath Dr. M.A. Rajalakshmi, whom I have interviewed in chapter four, has for example presented papers at the First National Conference on Autism organised by the Institute for Cognitive and Communicative Neurosciences (1999); the XII National Homeopathic Congress in Khajuraho (2001); the South Asian Regional Conference on Autism – Building Bridges (2008) organised by Action for Autism, India; the Global Autism Convention Bangalore (2011); and the 'Untangle Autism 2013' Conference Bahrain (2013).

Homeopaths tend to be invited by charities to speak about their methodology and approach to treating autism. Presentations will often include case studies to illustrate the changes before and after treatment. Self-treatment is not appropriate for ASD and it is always recommended to consult with a qualified professional homeopath. It is perhaps this lack of accessibility in a community where parents advise and share information between themselves that makes charities less inclined to promote homeopathy and nor would they want to be seen to be promoting a particular practitioner. For these reasons it is hard for homeopaths to interact with charities in giving specific training or guidance in the use of homeopathy.

Ursula Kraus-Harper, whom I have mentioned several times in this book, was invited to speak at the Treating Autism Conference September 2012 in the UK. This has helped to raise the profile of homeopathy within the UK autism community.

J.B. Handley, co-founder of Generation Rescue, Jenny McCarthy's autism organisation, felt sufficiently strongly about the benefits of homeopathic treatment that she wrote the following in the foreword to Dr. Tinus Smits' *Autism Beyond Despair – Cease Therapy* (Smits 2010, p.x):

> [The CEASE approach to treating autism] stands out among many others for its clarity, simplicity, and, perhaps most importantly, its focus on cause. The fact that it costs a fraction of some other therapies is a bonus and makes it accessible to parents staggering under the cost of treating their autistic child.

So perhaps homeopathy is worth investigating further!

CHAPTER NINE

THE MOST COMMONLY INDICATED HOMEOPATHIC TREATMENT STRATEGIES

Homeopathic materia medica – what this is and how it is applied. Homeopathic remedies. Discovering a few homeopathic remedies. Critique of different methodologies.

MOST COMMONLY INDICATED TREATMENT STRATEGIES

There are different ways in which a homeopath will commence treatment for the adult or child with a diagnosis of autism spectrum disorder (ASD).

The main strategies include:

- totality prescription: finding the 'similimum'

- 'never been well since' aetiology, for example a particular immunisation or other drug damage may be prescribed in potency

- examining family medical history, vitally important if born with problem

- addressing pregnancy or birth trauma – not only physical but also emotional

- support for damaged bowel flora

- single dose, multiple doses in series, liquid dose, LMs (50 millesimal potency).

All of these approaches or a combination of them give great flexibility in adjusting the strength of the prescription to the patient's individual susceptibility. And it is largely possible to avoid aggravations or side-effects when prescribing homeopathic remedies.

HOMEOPATHIC MATERIA MEDICA
What it is and how it is applied

I have used the exploration of various homeopathic remedy types in this chapter to demonstrate and illustrate a number of principles underpinning homeopathic thinking. The information given here on the homeopathic remedies is not sufficient to prescribe on, but simply presents elementary vignettes of the remedy discussed. There are numerous books available to the professional homeopath, and curious layperson, describing all of the homeopathic remedies in more detail. It is recommended that you visit a properly qualified homeopathic practitioner for a detailed case taking for your child and the careful selection of an individually chosen remedy.

First I explain how materia medica is collected and how it is applied. I will then look at some specific homeopathic remedies and how they are expressed in the ASD child.

Materia medica is the name given to the collated information on the action of homeopathic medicines or remedies. It is distinct from the pharmacology of the substances used, which only describes the constituents of the substance rather than its action. Drug action of homeopathic medicines is much broader in scope than that of conventional medications. It is expected that a homeopathic remedy will have an effect on all levels of the human organism, which is what makes it such a powerful and holistic form of therapy. There are three sources of materia medica: homeopathic clinical trial, known as a proving; toxicology and properties of the substance; and clinical experience.

'Homeopathic drug pictures' is a useful way of describing the information, as each remedy is described in terms of its effects on the emotions and intellectual aspects of a person; their reaction to foods, weather and temperature, their sleep and dreams and the various parts of the body – head, eyes, ears, nose, face, mouth, throat, appetite, stomach, food likes and dislikes, abdomen, stools, urinary organs, sexual organs, respiratory organs, chest, back, upper and lower limbs and skin. Although not every remedy will have an effect in all of these areas, effects across the whole of the system provide useful information to enable a closer match between patient and remedy to be made. Some symptoms indicative of disturbance or disease may have no apparent connection with the diagnosis of ASD but are characteristic of both the patient and the remedy.

Homeopathic drug trials are known as provings – the testing of a homeopathically prepared medicine on a healthy group of people. During a proving the participants are asked to note down all changes that they experience while taking the homeopathic remedy, for the following 30 days and at regular intervals thereafter, should any strong symptoms or patterns arise. At the end of this time the information from all of the participants is collected. This forms the basis of the initial remedy picture. Over time other symptoms may be added from clinical experience, and information from toxicology of the substance may also be incorporated into the materia medica. The potentised homeopathic remedy may have an opposite or different effect to a herbal remedy made from the same substance. For instance *Hypericum perfoliatum* is used homeopathically and herbally; however in homeopathy it is prescribed for damage to nerves, whereas herbally it is known as the popular herbal anti-depressant St. John's Wort.

How it is applied in practice

At the client's initial consultation information needs to be collected in depth, which will usually take one to two hours. As well as relying on observation and questioning of the patient themselves, especially in the case of a child, the homeopath will take note of information and observations from the parents or main caregivers. A full case taking has been conducted taking into account the patient's temperament, emotional expression, likes and dislikes, reactions to the external environment, sleep and dreams, fears, food likes and dislikes and so on, as well as a full medical history and top-to-toe body symptom questionnaire. This will be analysed according to homeopathic principles and a remedy selected which most closely matches the overall symptom picture of the patient. (The analysis is often done after the patient has left, and can take over an hour.)

Let us take a simple example to start with: if a child has a fever with red flushed cheeks, eyes with dilated pupils, a throbbing headache and is having mild hallucinations they might be prescribed the homeopathic remedy *Belladonna*, which is listed in the materia medica for this specific set of symptoms. Not only did the original provers experience these symptoms, but Bella Donna (beautiful lady)/atropine drops were used by Italian women of a bygone age to make their eyes dilate prior to attending a ball.

A condition in the ASD range is far more complex than this. If a child presented with destructive temper tantrums, had asthma and night sweats for example they might benefit from the homeopathic remedy *Tuberculinum*.

Important note: Please do not be tempted to self-prescribe on the basis of the information given in this chapter as there is no one remedy for one named condition and there are over 3000 homeopathic remedies to choose from.

HOMEOPATHIC REMEDIES

The repertory (Synthesis Treasure edition; Schroyens 2013) lists 67 homeopathic remedies under the heading 'Destructiveness', for example. The homeopathic prescription is based on the matching of the characteristic symptoms of the patient with the characteristic symptoms of the remedy.

As stated earlier, the homeopath analyses the case notes according to homeopathic principles. This means looking for, among other things, those symptoms which are characteristic of the patient rather than of the diagnostic label. Uncommon, strange, rare or peculiar symptoms are of more importance in the anamnesis than common symptoms of the diagnosis. For example stimming may be a common symptom of autism, but a fascination with spinning objects is less general and the fear of a mirror in the room may be even more uncommon. Likewise the food likes and dislikes, sleep patterns and temperature modalities are key to choosing the remedy, regardless of the diagnosis. These are known in homeopathy as 'physical general symptoms'.

I want to say a little more in general about what homeopathic remedies are made from. Contrary to common misunderstanding they are not herbal remedies or made exclusively from plants. Ever since the beginning of homeopathy, remedies have been made from plants, animal products, disease products, minerals and metals. The homeopathic remedies most often prescribed for ASD children might include substances such as potentised *Mercury*, *Barium carbonicum* (both of which are chemical elements), *Carcinosin* and *Tuberculinum* (which are potentised human disease products), *Stramonium* and *Hyoscymus* (potentised toxic plants) and *Bufo* (potentised toad); so homeopathic remedies are not all nice plants. All remedies are safe to take because of the way they are prepared; and homeopaths always match the symptom pattern to the patient, regardless of what it was made from.

Homeopaths work according to a number of definite principles (which are defined in the glossary) and will take these into account in their interpretation of what is going on with each patient who they meet and select an individual remedy for:

- the vital force or disease on a dynamic level

- individual susceptibility

- the law of similars

- provings

- potentisation

- Hering's law of cure

- miasmatic theory.

DISCOVERING A FEW HOMEOPATHIC REMEDIES

Agaricus

This remedy will be indicated in boisterous (along with 162 other homeopathic remedies), lively children who are silly, sing and laugh without reason, make up verses or poems, embrace and kiss freely. They will be clumsy and awkward. They are likely to have facial tics, grimace and jerk. The skin is the area of the body that is often affected by this remedy and may itch or burn, feel cold in spots and have redness looking like frostbite or chilblains. Father Christmas could almost be seen as an adult Agaricus with his hilarity, laughing without reason, kissing and embracing strangers and his frostbitten extremities. *Agaricus* is one of the homeopathic remedies that is indicated for children who are late in learning to walk, talk and in general learning development; they will make mistakes in speech and writing and are very likely to suffer with some kind of convulsive movement.

Baryta carbonicum

The child requiring this remedy will be timid and shy; often hiding behind the parent or the furniture. Kim Elia (2012) says that a presentation of this remedy in autism that he sees in practice is 'Need support to stand due to lack of muscle tone. Head falls to side. Does not recognise anything.' He also says that they 'cannot be aggressive, will not fight back, reproaches self and apologetic'. The remedy type is certainly well known for its indecision and lack of self-confidence. They seem to have a tremendous need for support expressed in the idea that he is walking on his knees! One child patient of mine, aged seven, expressed this as a need for protection by God. They commonly feel that they are being laughed at and mocked or that people are talking about them. Physically this remedy will often be considered due to the hypertrophy of the tonsils or other swollen glands. They may have offensive perspiration of the feet, like another remedy *Silica*, which is also lacking in self-confidence. Like *Tuberculinum* they also have a tendency for recurrent colds, but the character is obviously very different. The child requiring a prescription of the homeopathic remedy *Baryta carbonicum* is likely to be small and dwarfish or to grow slowly. When choosing to prescribe the homeopathic remedy *Baryta carbonicum*, it is also important to consider the similar but slightly different salts of *Baryta muriaticum, Baryta phosphoricum* or *Baryta sulphuricum*. The American homeopaths, Judyth Reichenberg-Ullman, Robert Ullman and Ian Luepker in their book (2005 pp.74–76, 133), discuss cases which responded to *Barya sulphuricum* and *Baryta phosphoricum*.

Bufo

Pharmacology: *Bufo* is prepared from the poison expressed from the skin glands of a toad, which is then potentised homeopathically. This may seem a strange substance to use; however Italian endocrinologists (Emanuele *et al.* 2010) found in their study that 'elevated urine levels of the endogenous psychotomimetic molecule bufotenine may play a role in ASD and schizophrenia, and can be correlated with hyperactivity scores in autism'. The homeopathic proving of *Bufo* by Mure in 1840 is referred to in Allen's Encyclopedia (1990, p.318) and its clinical use predates this by 170 years. Various toxicological effects had been noted in people who came into contact with the skin of the toad and carrying out a homeopathic proving of this substance (see glossary) produced a range of mental, emotional and physical symptoms which have been seen to match the symptom picture of many ASD children. The child requiring a homeopathic prescription of *Bufo* would typically exhibit a desire for solitude, when they are on their own they will often masturbate excessively; they may be intelligent in a narrow field (be very knowledgeable about a particular subject) yet have delayed development in general. They tend to have an overdeveloped large physical body and an underdeveloped childish mind. They can be prone to destructive anger and become angry when not understood. They may have convulsions during sleep.

Cannabis indica

A number of American homeopaths have written about the usefulness of this homeopathic remedy in working with ASD children including Kim Elia (2012 webinar). There may have been a history of drug use in the parents at some point which has become engrafted onto either the child at conception or in utero or perhaps even pre-conception. Philippa Fibert (2012, pp.15–17) also refers to this in her article 'Nature or nurture? what drives the rise in behavioural disorders and her Consecutive Case Series (Fibert 2014). Other social drugs taken to excess or in a sensitive or susceptible individual may need to be prescribed in their homeopathic form. As individuals we do not exist in isolation and it may be that the need for the prescription of this homeopathic remedy and *Carcinosin* below is a reflection of the times in which we live.

Carcinosin

Patients can be worried by the idea of taking this remedy, made from potentised breast cancer cells, but like all homeopathic nosodes (see glossary) beyond the dilution of 6× there remains no physical trace of the substance; but rather an energetic or bioelectrical imprint of the substance, a dynamically prepared remedy works on a dynamic level. There are several well documented cases of children who have benefited tremendously from this homeopathic remedy. The most well documented case with long-term follow up is the case of Max, who is written about by his mother – Amy Lansky – in her excellent book *Impossible Cure* (2003). Roberto Petrucci has also shown video follow up of a child who benefited from the same remedy at his international seminars and refers to this remedy and its 'incredible action' in his excellent book *Children Homeopathic Materia Medica with Repertorial Symptoms* (Petrucci 2007). As with *Tuberculinum*, another homeopathic nosode, a family history of a particular disease can be indicative of the need for a homeopathic nosode to clear the inherited miasm. However, most homeopaths tend to prescribe not on a theoretical application of this idea but rather on a clear symptom picture of the remedy. Not everyone who has had a parent or grandparent with cancer will require the homeopathic remedy *Carcinosin*. Although family history is one symptom that would be taken into account in choosing to prescribe this remedy, other major indications would be a lack of normal childhood diseases and fever or a very severe case of one of the childhood diseases. It is suggested by some medical philosophers that childhood fevers and indeed childhood diseases are an important part of developing the immature immune system's own ability to respond. This might in some way go towards explaining why this remedy is so frequently indicated when childhood fevers are constantly suppressed by Tylenol and Calpol and childhood illness countered by an extensive program of immunisation.

Helium

Jan Scholten (1996) in his book *Homeopathy and the Elements* postulates that this remedy could be good for helping people with autism to be more present in the world:

> Autism is a very appropriate word for Helium. They don't feel like entering this world. They prefer to stay in themselves to experience their own being. They are not interested in finding out about values and meaning in life. They don't feel any affinity with those matters, they simply live. They have gone through the process of incarnation, they accept they are here and they don't doubt that fact. But they don't want to be involved in the why and wherefores of their existence. Their behaviour makes it very difficult to understand for other people. You can't get a grip on them, as if they are slipping away through your fingers each time you try and establish contact. This can be seen in autistic children. They won't let you come near. You can do what you like with them, they simply won't react. They remain locked up inside themselves, unapproachable and distant. (p.95)

Sherr (2013) in his book on Helium writes:

> Many provers felt a strong desire to be alone and undisturbed, and yearned for peace and quiet. They found a variety of ways to avoid company and to cut themselves off from the world, often hiding behind a book or shutting all the doors and windows. Many provers experienced an intense aversion to talking, touching or engaging in any social interaction, with a definite aversion to talking on the telephone. The feeling was one of 'leave me alone, I don't need or want anyone'. This isolation was often accompanied by apathy. The Helium patient may seem introverted, cold and distant to others. The sense of separation might manifest as a calm tranquillity, as if not affected or touched by anything. A feeling of living in one's own world, calm, relaxed and not bothered by external circumstances. (p.42)

The homeopathic preparation of Helium was first written about by Jan Scholten (1996) and proved by Jeremy Sherr in 1995 and published in 2013, so it is a new homeopathic remedy. Searching the internet using the terms 'homeopathy helium' produces two encouraging parent stories, especially on the blog 'Boy connected – improving Dante's health and wellbeing using the CEASE homeopathic protocol along with others'. The post entitled 'Helium rocks' (Dante's mom 2012) has particularly powerful photographs of Dante when he was on medication for seizures and when homeopathy reduced the seizures.

Dante's mother observed these changes when her son began taking Helium:

- more energy – this was the most notable change, the day after the first dose

- seizure fluctuations (some were stronger episodes) accompanied by a rapid decline in seizure frequency, reaching *zero* in two weeks

- much more physical strength (probably benefited from the decline in seizures)

- no drooling

- great stability on his feet

- great interest in the world around him

- he's back to making his wishes understood, using PECs (Picture Exchange System), signs, and approximating words

- he's very loving and appreciative – giving hugs and kisses all around

- interested in other's (different) foods

- very healthy.

The healing journey was started with the Modified Atkins Diet and the turnaround happened with homeopathy.

Helleborus

It is interesting that the main toxic constituent of the plant Hellebore is Hellebrin, which is chemically identical to bufadienolide discussed in relation to the remedy *Bufo*, although I am not aware of any similar research with this substance. The person requiring this remedy, even when there is no actual physical or nerve damage to the sensory organs of sight and hearing, has great difficulty in receiving communication and appears somewhat stupefied. If they are asked a question they will reflect for a long time before answering, and may need the question to be repeated. They are forgetful of what they have heard, said or read and their speech is slow. Physically they may have a constant chewing motion of the jaw, roll their head from side to side, bore their heads into the pillow at night and may strike or grasp their head with their hands They may be spoon biters: *Helleborus* is one of only ten remedies listed in the Synthesis 10.5 Treasure Edition repertory (Schroyens 2013) for this.

Hyoscymus

The prescriber will be led to this remedy by the intense sibling jealousy exhibited by this child. There may be shamelessness, high sexuality, loquacity and malice. Their rages are very aggressive, biting and striking others, and they may turn to self-harm. They can be abusive and express feelings of absolute hatred. On a physical level there are likely to be muscular twitches and convulsions.

Lanthanides

The strange sounding group of homeopathic remedies are made from the chemical elements numbers 57–70, which are very much part of everyday life in the 21st century. They have strong magnetic qualities so are used in tiny electric motors and as magnets in headphones. They are used in the manufacture and components of CDs, colour televisions, self-cleaning ovens, film industry lighting, cigarette lighters, as catalysts in the petroleum industry, in lasers and ceramics and in many more modern everyday goods.

Since the beginning of homeopathy over 200 years ago and Hahnemann's original work with *Arsenicum* and *Mercury*, homeopaths have studied toxic substances in our environment and considered how they might be impacting on the human species both as a whole and individually. The work to date with the *Lanthanide* remedies has been quite theoretical, with some clinical experience. These remedies have been used more in Europe than the rest of the world, but may well hold the key for some sufferers from ASD. Welte and Kuntosch state that:

> The *Lanthanides* are also good candidates to treat autism spectrum disorders. Their remedy picture shows an excessive self-centeredness but at a more complex self-reflective level than the *Lithium salts*, who react more spontaneously and are more childishly egocentric. The experience in our practice is that both the *Lithium salts* and the *Lanthanides* are well indicated for autistic disorders and can achieve a lot. The *Lithium* personalities seem to be helplessly at the mercy of their disorder, which runs right through them, whereas the

Lanthanides are maybe more able to recognise their disturbance and reflect on it. *Lithium* is more impulsive, whereas the *Lanthanides* appear to be more accessible at the intellectual level. In addition, the Lanthanides are especially effective for reading and writing difficulties. (2010 p.18)

Lycopodium

The *Lycopodium* child will dominate the home, being dictatorial and bossy with a love of power over others. A remedy can sometimes be understood by looking at the name, for example *Lycopodium*, like (to be on) a podium (position of intellectual power). They will have a strong intellect but weak body. They will be particularity prone to gastrointestinal complaints. In clinical practice the remedy can be mistaken for *Tuberculinum*. They might be the proverbial 'angel at school, devil at home'.

Mercurius

This remedy's usefulness in the homeopathic treatment of ASD is possibly partly due to the effect of mercury poisoning from *Thimerosal* contained in many immunisations, which has overloaded the system. Formaldehyde, which is also used in vaccines, is a mercury derivative. It is interesting that a homeopathic preparation of Aluminium which is another component of many vaccines, is rarely prescribed for ASD children; it is in fact a more common prescription for elderly people. This again underlines the point that homeopathic prescriptions are based on the principle of matching symptom pictures between the remedy and the individual. Although the Japanese homeopath, Toraki Yui, uses homeopathic *Mercurius* as standard in cases of developmental disorder, CEASE therapists and others are more likely to use MMR in homeopathic form or any other vaccine in homeopathic form if a child has obviously never been well since a certain immunisation. The homeopathic remedy *Mercurius* is more likely to be prescribed on the basis of an overall symptom picture.

Opium

There will often be a history of a severe fright in cases requiring this remedy and a stupefied, besotted look. There may well be inactivity of the bowel or its opposite diarrhoea. The sense impression of or a flashback to a previous fright may re-occur frequently. The related drug *Pethidine* is sometimes required as a prescription for young children. *Pethidine* is used as a painkilling drug, as well as an anti-spasmodic; it is often used during labour and crosses the placenta. It is a synthetic version of morphine, another opiate. Essentially having experienced trauma in the past, the patient requiring a homeopathic dose of *Opium* will have become numb to allowing themselves further feelings that would remind them of previous painful experiences.

Stramonium

Children needing this remedy may experience fear and terror when they are alone and in the dark. They may be violent or the victim of some type of violence, and the remedy is often indicated after a particularly traumatic birth experience. I have frequently seen the inner experience of the *Stramonium* child expressed in drawing with images of daggers, zombies and being cut in two. Their inner feeling is as if they are alone in the wilderness and about to be eaten by wild animals. There is often something quite appealing about them as they reach out to you and do not hide their inner feelings, although they are obviously deeply disturbed.

Ritualistic behaviour is often deployed, unconsciously, as protection from the inner sense of terror and fear of being injured.

Thuja

The choice of this remedy will take into account a mental rigidity or fixed ideas. There is likely to be a history of warty growths and a greasy skin. There is a marked sense of separation between mind/soul and body in the *Thuja* patient, they tend to hide their true selves from the world and often have a feeling that if anyone knew what they were like inside they would not like them, that they are ugly inside. This could be seen in the child making an effort to fit in to the expected norms of school behaviour for example. It can frequently develop when moving home or school, but a child can also just be born that way. They may have the feeling that there is someone standing beside them, an expression of the inner disconnectedness that they feel. There may be a sense that they are not fully in their body, a problem of incarnation perhaps depending on your spiritual world view. This can be expressed as a feeling of fragility, that they could easily break; the sense of someone beside them and their sense of separation within themselves.

Tuberculinum

The symptoms presented by the child requiring a prescription of the homeopathic remedy *Tuberculinum*, might include ritualistic behaviour, a strong fear of dogs; desires for fatty food, cold milk, smoked foods; and a tendency to catch repeated colds. They may well be allergic to animal fur and dander. Depending on where the child is on the autism spectrum there will be a different expression of the remedy. The destructiveness can be expressed as a malicious streak where not only will they break things during a tantrum, but they will break your favourite things. In children requiring other homeopathic remedies the destructiveness is usually a lot milder. They are often restless children with a desire to run away. Twenty-three other remedies are also listed in the Homeopathic Synthesis Repertory (2010) for the impulse to run away, so you cannot prescribe on one symptom alone, but always on the whole symptom picture. For example, contrast with other homeopathic remedy types, such as *Pulsatilla* or *Bismuth*, who will want to constantly hold the mother's hand. You will often see a Tubercular family history in previous generations which comes through to expression in the child with an effect on lungs, skin and glands; emaciation and night sweats. The child requiring the homeopathic remedy *Tuberculinum* is likely to grind their teeth and wet the bed during the night; but again 154 remedies are listed for involuntary urination at night (Schroyens 2013); underlining the importance of not taking any symptom in isolation or prescribing on the basis of one symptom alone.

CONCLUSION

In this chapter I have only looked at 14 homeopathic remedies. There are more than 3500 homeopathic remedies to choose from, so this brief discussion is merely an illustrative example, rather than an exploration of all the homeopathic remedies that would need to be considered in treating a patient on the autism spectrum. By describing these remedies I have clarified that the homeopathic prescription, or selection of the appropriate remedy, is not based on interpretation or observations of the emotional nature of the child alone, but also on very definite observable physical symptoms. There are homeopathic remedies that will address the full range of the autism spectrum from high functioning to severe autism with accompanying convulsions or epilepsy.

CRITIQUE OF METHODOLOGIES

Classical homeopathy

It is possible that this approach may not address maintaining causes or toxicity. There is anecdotal evidence that heavy metal toxicity can reduce dramatically after a well-chosen remedy, but it would be pertinent to see some research around this. The value of diet alongside homeopathy has been discussed elsewhere in the book.

The rubrics in the homeopathic repertory (see glossary) can be inadequate because they are predominantly based on what comes up in provings rather than verified clinical symptoms. Sometimes a remedy can be included on too little poorly verified information, so there is a danger of over- or under-valuation of symptoms included.

The practitioner needs to have studied the way in which each particular remedy presents in autism spectrum disorder. Kim Elia (2012) has done some good work around this.

The road to improvement can be long and winding with zig zagging from one remedy to another, but with persistence and patience on the part of both homeopath and parents/carers results can, in my experience, be remarkable.

Finding the *similimum*, the most similar remedy for a patient, can take time. There are potentially an infinite number of substances which could be the particular similimum for an individual.

Fortunately there are remedies which are indicated more frequently in any condition and a similar enough remedy can benefit a patient enormously. As the interviews, the overview of the literature and the chapters contributed by Simon Taffler and Linlee Jordan show, there are a group of remedies which are frequently indicated and work well for patients with ASD. However, a limitation of the classical homeopathic approach is that it is possible to prescribe a remedy that has some effect and is close to the similimum, but a more accurately matching remedy searched for with perseverance on the part of both the parent or patient and the homeopath can achieve far more remarkable results.

CEASE Therapy (Compete Elimination of Autistic Spectrum Expression)

CEASE therapy is a homeopathic approach to working with children on the autism spectrum, which many parents will have heard of and practitioners are using. As a new system it may not having the backing of a solid enough experiential background. I would personally like to see more published about the use of this therapy by practitioners who are using it exclusively in their practices. Practitioners might make assertive claims about its efficacy after having only undertaken a short training in this approach, in addition to their homeopathic qualification, but with little experience with it in practice. There are also, though, many very experienced homeopaths who are incorporating it into their practices.

It can be a doorway into the world of homeopathy for many parents, as it is easier to understand than the classical homeopathic approach. It appears closer to allopathic or conventional medical thinking in that 'same' is used to treat 'same', and this is an easier concept for people to embrace than the idea of treating with 'similars' on which classical homeopathy is based.

CEASE was developed by the Dutch homeopath, Tinus Smits. He worked with over 300 children with an autism diagnosis before his untimely death in 2010. CEASE therapy is a combination of classical homeopathy and isotherapy. Homeopathic remedies treat 'like with like' – a substance that can cause similar symptoms is used to treat the patient's symptoms, whereas isopathy means treating 'same with same'. Isopathy prescribes the same substance that seemed to have triggered the initial decline in health. The aim of this is to detoxify substances that caused a decline in health or an apparent onset of autistic traits.

Perhaps surprisingly, Tinus Smits and those who have worked with his system have found that many substances, which are often not considered toxic in themselves, have proved just too much for the individual susceptibility of the child to tolerate. An already overloaded or damaged immune system reaches breaking point. These substances and whether they are or are not considered causative factors by the scientific community remains controversial. However, in clinical practice it is often observed that there is an improvement in health following the administration of these substances in isopathic form. Detoxes can be quite extreme in some cases and there can often be a return of previously experienced symptoms in the healing process. This is essentially in line with Hering's law, a cornerstone of homeopathic philosophy, which states that disturbance moves from above downwards, from innermost organs to outermost organs and from top to bottom of the body. However, the rigidity of the CEASE protocol with its repetition of frequent doses perhaps sometimes needs to be tailored more sensitively to the patient's individual sensitivity.

The very name of the therapy is controversial, as there is ongoing debate both within the autism community and elsewhere, as to whether autism is a psychological diagnosis, a disease that is treatable or a different way of being with its own associated problems and advantages. However, homeopaths are realists and their aim is to work with the symptoms presented by a patient. The troublesome symptoms of autism that might be helped using CEASE and other homeopathic approaches include: lack of eye contact, communication problems including levels of speech and interaction with others, inability to eat a range of foods, hyperactivity and hypersensitivity and associated medical problems that the child or adult might have. There is obviously the need for more research and clinical audit to back up these anecdotal claims. I achieve results in the following areas in my practice using classical homeopathy alone, so deciding whether CEASE therapy or pure classical homeopathy is the better approach is still open to question.

However, many homeopaths worldwide are likely to use some detox/isopathic prescriptions at some stage in the treatment of patients on the autism spectrum. They may not necessarily follow the CEASE protocol in doing so.

It can take a long time and much trial and error to find the apparent causal factor which needs to be antidoted to restore the system to a healthier functioning. If the practitioner prescribes the substance early on in treatment, since when symptoms first developed, results in some cases can be dramatic. In other cases it seems necessary to work through a lot of substances until perhaps finding the needle in the haystack, for example the hair dye that the mother used in pregnancy. Classical homeopathy prescribes on the symptoms presented by the patient so does not involve the same requirement to find the incriminating substance.

In my experience, parents, and others are often not aware of all the drugs that they have taken over a period of time.

I personally dislike following a protocol. It seems to me that there can be very difficult exacerbations of symptoms from the use of this method, which can be difficult for the patient and the family to go through.

However, both Philippa Fibert and Ursula Kraus-Harper, two prominent UK homeopaths working with this therapy in their practices, have seen this approach work very well for their patients. Certainly there is a strong argument for prescribing a dose or more of the substance to which symptoms seem to date back; and many homeopaths will, for example, include potentised vaccines at some point in their treatment plan, often when the action of other remedies appears to come to a standstill.

The isopathic component of CEASE therapy alone may not offer the other constitutional benefits of homeopathy such as improved immunity and resistance to colds and other acute infections; however, when combined with classical homeopathy this is potentially possible.

During the course of writing this book I have spoken with many parents and practitioners who have used this approach who have reported significant changes in their children or children they have been working with using the CEASE approach.

Philippa Fibert (2012, p.16) writes of her observational case study of a group of 20 children with a diagnosis of ADHD, four of whom had a diagnosis of ASD, that 'responses to being given homeopathic preparations of these toxins [smoking cigarettes or cannabis during pregnancy, on the contraceptive pill when becoming pregnant, on Clozapine when pregnant, working in a launderette when pregnant, multiple courses of antibiotics, MMR vaccination] in ascending potencies were dramatic'.

Complex homeopathy

This is when a mixture of potentised medicines is prescribed for a condition. This does not follow the principles of homeopathy, matching the remedy to the individual patient, and is generally not approved of by professionally qualified homeopaths. It tends to be self-prescribed and is sold over the internet without a consultation.

Support for damaged bowel flora

During homeopathic treatment some homeopaths will use remedies such as *Gaertner* and *Saccharum officinalle* to support the digestive process homeopathically, others will expect the individually selected constitutional remedies to act on the system as a whole.

Danny Dushan Ron has written about the results that he is achieving with intercurrent doses of his *Candida Mix*, in-between doses of the individually selected similimum prescription.

CHAPTER TEN

RESEARCH AND
PROFESSIONAL RECOGNITION

*Complementary and alternative medicine research
and integration into healthcare. Professional recognition.
Funding treatment. Funding research. The future.*

From the outset homeopathy has been a controversial therapeutic modality which can be hard to understand. My intention in this book has been to show that homeopathy has a role to play in the management of autism spectrum disorder (ASD). There is a constant swing, it seems, between including homeopathy and other non-conventional systems of medical care in a vision of integrated healthcare, and at other times vigorous attempts to discredit it entirely. In some countries it forms a large part of the health service, for example one in four prescriptions in France are homeopathic; in other countries it is very much marginalised. In some countries only doctors can practice homeopathy, in others it is also practised by professional homeopaths. The setting in which homeopathy finds itself raises problems of professional recognition. However, many countries have a number of registers of homeopaths who have been through a comprehensive education in homeopathy and agree to abide by a Code of Ethics and Practice. A list of national homeopathic organisations in Australia, the US and the UK is included in the resources section of the book in the appendix. Personal recommendation is often the way in which a practitioner is chosen. Homeopathy has a good safety record and is generally regarded as being without side-effects. Depending on where you live, the fees for a homeopathic consultation will vary and may or may not be met by a health insurance scheme. Due to the relatively marginal position of homeopathy, research is not well funded. Although homeopathy is said to be the second most used form of healthcare in the world by the World Health Organisation (2005), the largest numbers of users are in less wealthy countries. In India over a million people are said to depend solely on homeopathy, while in the UK 15 per cent of the population have said they use it and rely on its health benefits.

The multi-national pharmaceutical companies fund the majority of medical research worldwide; they have little interest in homeopathy, although they may perceive it as a threat to the uptake of conventional drug regimes and attempt to discredit it. There is also little motivation for pharmaceutical companies to fund homeopathic research as they are not generally involved in the distribution of homeopathic remedies or their licensing and the profits to be made are much smaller than in conventional medicine.

The individualised nature of homeopathic treatment does not readily lend itself to randomised control trials (RCTs), which is the standard by which the effectiveness of medicines is currently judged. Even so, of the 163 RCTs in homeopathy more have been positive (67) than negative (11) (Find a Homeopath 2013). RCTs are seen as the gold standard for proof of medical efficacy. There are many published case reports worldwide and a number of small pieces of qualitative research into the effectiveness of homeopathy as a therapeutic intervention in ASD, which are worth reading to form your own opinion. Many of these have been referred to in this book.

There are strong arguments for evaluating a therapy according to its effectiveness as opposed to its efficacy. Effectiveness studies use real-world clinicians and clients who have multiple diagnoses or needs. Effective treatment provides positive results in a practice. In contrast, efficacious treatment provides positive results in a controlled experimental research trial. A study that shows a treatment approach to be efficacious means that the study produced good outcomes, which were identified in advance, in a controlled experimental trial. Case reports are sometimes dismissed as being merely anecdotal by homeopathy's detractors, however, they can be considered of value from an effectiveness viewpoint as can the patient evaluation tool, Measure Yourself Medical Outcome Profile (MYMOP). There have been a number of projects within the homeopathic community where video footage has been used to demonstrate the effectiveness of treatment and this certainly has the potential to demonstrate changes in behaviour over a period of time. Perhaps video evidence is the way forward for parental acceptance of homeopathy, even if it will not satisfy the scientific community.

Frei (2006) in his paper on a long-term study on attention deficit hyperactivity disorder (ADHD) raised a number of problems for homeopathic research; as he saw it, successful prescription

> depends upon precise observations by the patient or parents and the initial phase of treatment is often characterised by the use of different medications until an optimal response is reached. The effectiveness of homeopathy, in which the active substance is no longer traceable due to its high dilution, is contested... The need for individually prescribed homeopathic medication complicates the planning of a double blind trial. (p.4)

Frei gets round this by blinding only after the correct individual medication for each patient has been found; deterioration was then studied under placebo.

In my interview with Philippa Fibert (2013), quoted in Chapter four, she states that in her opinion, 'one of the main issues preventing the recognition of homeopathy's role in treating autism spectrum disorder is the lack of comparative research in peer reviewed journals'. Referring to the question of efficacy versus effectiveness she replied that she would like to see:

> Pragmatic effectiveness trials (as opposed to placebo controlled efficacy trials) where the totality of the homeopathic intervention is compared to treatment as usual.

I would like to build a great big cohort of children with ASD and randomly select different groups to try the different therapies that parents are trying, including homeopathy, to see which are more effective. This is what I hope to do once I've finished my PhD…

When I asked Carol Boyce (2013) what kind of research she would like to see, to show the effectiveness of treating these children with homeopathy, she replied as follows (see pp.69–70 of this volume):

There is already a body of research showing the potential of homeopathy – hundreds of case reports that have been analysed, some pilot studies, albeit limited in their scope, have shown significant results. But we need studies which can test homeopathy, in the way that it is meant to be practiced. I believe it's both possible and urgent to develop studies that allow both the individualization of prescriptions and a double blind arm. My own work with a pilot study has been a long and difficult road without even contemplating the funding required to run the study. Despite the involvement of a respected university department and a very experienced lead investigator (100+ published papers – all in conventional medicine) signed onto the project, we could not get the proposal through the Internal Review Body's ethical board. Not because they were afraid the homeopathic medicines might harm the children, but because there was: 'No evidence in the medical literature showing that homeopathy is useful in the treatment of ASD' and therefore they did not feel comfortable approving a pilot study into the possibility that homeopathy might be useful in the treatment of ASD. The board also wanted the exact prescription and posology for each of the children submitted before approval could be considered, and once the study began the protocols could not be changed. Of course this is like asking a sprinter to race in the Olympic finals wearing wellington boots. The sprinter will finish the race but they won't be able to demonstrate anywhere near their full potential! It was very difficult to explain the principles of individualised medicine. It would have been easier if we had named a medicine and a potency and dosage that we intended to put on the market at some point in the future. That we wanted to test a system, rather than a marketable product was difficult for the board to fathom and as science contracts rather than expands, it was too much of a 'risk' – not for the children who might have been helped, but for the university and its reputation. It's been an instructive process so far and if I didn't know beforehand how difficult it is to get homeopathic research even onto the starting blocks, I do now.

The founder of homeopathy, Samuel Hahnemann (1921), defined disease as a dynamic disturbance which needed to be cured dynamically in Aphorism 9. I have referred to this rather loosely as 're-balancing the system'. Homeopathy is often criticised by its detractors for being unscientific and therefore not possible – or nothing better than placebo. The placebo argument is frequently raised against homeopathy, however, it is used for babies, young children and animals and they don't need to 'believe' that it will work for it to do so. There is much research on veterinary homeopathy and a number of key pieces of research on homeopathy for children's health complaints; but it is beyond the scope of this book to discuss these in more depth.

It has long been held that there is an electromagnetic component to homeopathy. William A. Tiller of Stanford University (1981) in his Foreword to George Vithoulkas's book *The Science of Homeopathy* (1986, pp.xi–xiv) refers to this electromagnetic component. Since then we have had Benveniste *et al.*'s paper (1991) on the memory of water, for which he was sadly ridiculed, and most recently the noble prize winner, Professor Luc Montagnier and colleagues' papers on the electromagnetic properties of water (2009, 2011). Speaking of homeopathy he said 'High dilutions of something are not nothing. They are water structures which mimic the original molecules. It is not pseudoscience. It's not quackery. These are real phenomena which deserve further study' (Montagnier 2010).

Further recent hypotheses in the field of advanced physics refer to the possibility of a nanoparticle effect or the effects of Quantum Coherence Domains. It seems that high dilutions emit an electromagnetic signal that can be detected, recorded and played back. There is much excellent information on the Homeopathic Research Institute's website and also in the research section of the Society of Homeopaths' UK website. This is all important as homeopathy has had an ongoing battle to be accepted by the conventional medical world since its inception; and it is possible that quantum physics will one day explain the method through which homeopathy functions. However, in the meantime, we have to rely upon the research and evidence of effectiveness, observed in the clinical setting, in numerous clinical audits and papers referred to in this book and available elsewhere. However, as many users of homeopathy would say 'homeopathy worked for me'.

The Swiss health authorities commissioned a Health Technology Assessment (Bornhöft and Matthiessen 2012) report on 'effectiveness, appropriateness, safety and costs of homeopathy in healthcare'. The report was commissioned by them to inform decision making on the further inclusion of homeopathy in the list of services covered by statutory health insurance in Switzerland. It confirmed homeopathy as 'a valuable addition to the conventional medical landscape – a status it has been holding for a long time in practical healthcare'.

As many of the contributors to this book have stated, there is a need for research, and funding for that research. However, more is happening, such as the Homeopathic Research Institute's 2012 Barcelona Conference 'Cutting Edge Research in Homeopathy'.

Conventional medicine has little to offer in terms of real deep change for the child with autism, the costs of providing healthcare is rising worldwide with major funding issues in the UK and US. Thailand has made the decision to support the implementation of complementary and alternative medicine into the health system, as they see that the country would be bankrupted by following the US or UK conventional drug-based approach. Belgian homeopaths have been invited to advise the Ministry of Health in Thailand (Schroyens and Hamilton 2012, p.6). Much discussion goes on in the European Parliament about complementary healthcare. In June 2013 there was a 'Complementary and Alternative Medicine: An Investment in Health' conference held in the European Parliament. The European Commissioner for Health and Consumer Policy, Tonio Borg (2013), stated that:

> It is an important principle of the [European] Union's pharmaceutical legislation that patients should have access to the medicinal products of their choice. This includes innovative medicines as much as traditional herbal and homeopathic medicinal products... Patients often know what treatment works for them, and which healthcare is efficient for their condition. This can include complementary medicine. (2013, pp.3–6)

So in choosing to use homeopathy, you are following your European, at least, 'constitutional' rights! Homeopathy is still recognised by the UK government and has been part of the National Health Service (NHS) since its inception in 1948.

CHAPTER ELEVEN

HOW HOMEOPATHY ENHANCES THE GIFT OF ASD

The gift of ASD. Homeopathy's role in managing aggression, enhancing wellbeing and improving physical health. Finding a role in society.

I remember being very moved when I first saw a TV documentary about Temple Grandin's (2005) book *Animals in Translation* and how her particular view of the world had made a profound difference to animal welfare in American slaughterhouses. I am sure her journey has not been an easy one and it would be patronising on my part to comment on the 'gift of ASD' for anyone else; it is for the individuals to speak for themselves.

The neurodiversity or autism rights movement sees autism as a different way of thinking and interacting with the world, rather than a disability. Autistic UK (ARM) seeks to represent people with neurodiversity in the UK; in the US the organisations are the Autistic Self-Advocacy Network and Autism Network International. As a practitioner I have always tried to understand the way that a child perceives the world and recognise that society, most particularly education, needs to change its response to the message that these children can bring to us. Jim Sinclair (1993) in his essay 'Don't Mourn for Us' accused parents who long to cure their children's autism of really hoping 'that one day we will cease to be, strangers you can love will move in behind our faces'.

However in many of the children that I have met, there have been difficulties with some of the symptoms associated with their gift. Controlling aggression and anger for example can be a real problem in many families with ASD children. Not only can sibling rivalry or violence to brothers and sisters be amplified, but also there is often a marked level of violence to primary caregivers. This is something that in my experience, and that of many other homeopaths, can be helped significantly with homeopathy. I have had cases of children that have banged their heads against the wall, hit themselves, or assaulted their parents. Violence to parents may be very extreme on occasions. The successful selection and prescription of a homeopathic remedy has, in my experience, resolved this behaviour quickly. At the start of treatment this type of behaviour might re-occur and require repetition of the remedy. Over the course of treatment this behaviour ceases to be part of the picture. Although there may still be many challeneges for these children, homeopathic treatment enables them to be less of a danger to themselves and others.

As many of today's ASD children grow into adolescence and adulthood it becomes essential for both the safety of themselves and others that they are able to manage any violent impulses they have; and much better to do so in a way that does not involve medication with unknown or unpleasant side-effects. Even when the violence is not physically expressed it will often be noted in the dreams or language of the child; whether this indicates a response to some psychological traumas, or is a reaction to toxic damage to the brain or overload, cannot always be verified with certainty. However, aggression is frequently present in children with a diagnosis of ASD in my experience and it can be helped significantly with homeopathy; this is not only verified anecdotally but also in many of the small-scale research projects which I have previously referred to.

Homeopathy's role in improving physical health problems is significant. I recall the case of a six-year-old boy with autism who suffered from recurrent sore throats and was consequently missing many days of school. He was helped immensely by homeopathy in many ways, and now rarely suffers a day's illness. If a child is already finding the school environment difficult, having large amounts of time away from school with physical ill health is not going to help the situation. Both the conclusions of research projects from around the world, and personal experience, bear out the benefit to be gained from homeopathic treatment in managing toileting needs for example, whether it be incontinence or simply the need for extra assistance in managing this everyday task.

Finding a role in society is a rather ambitious topic to explore; I am sure that we all hope for our children that they will find lasting friendships, satisfying relationships, worthwhile occupations and happiness in their life choices. A survey by Autistic UK 2014 suggests that:

> At least one in every one hundred UK citizens is autistic, this may be a conservative estimate; this means that there are 600,000 or more autistic people living in the UK: 85 per cent are not in full-time employment, 66 per cent are not working at all, 60 per cent rely on their family for financial support, 33 per cent have not income at all. About 75 per cent have no friends or find it very difficult to make friends while 72 per cent would like to spend more time in the company of other people, only 14 per cent live independently. Over 70 per cent of those who do live independently have experienced bulling or harassment.

Carol Boyce (2010, p.16) suggests that 'one third of children diagnosed with ASD will never live independent lives, hold employment, have relationships or children of their own'. There can be no doubt that, whatever the percentages, we live in the age of an epidemic profoundly affecting our children and their chance to live a fulfilling life. Many families are torn apart by the challenge of living with, and loving these children, while managing their behaviour. I believe that homeopathy is a vital tool to help these children and their parents/carers, alongside other treatment modalities such as nutrition and speech therapy. I hope that this book has given you as a parent or carer the interest and knowledge to explore homeopathic treatment for your child. I would like to have given other healthcare professionals a greater understanding of homeopathy, to be able to confidently recommend it to families as a worthwhile avenue to explore. I intended to give homeopaths the confidence to understand the condition, and to appreciate other approaches that patients might be using, as well as greater confidence in managing their cases and clarity about the expectations of treatment. Most of all, my vision is that the information you have read in this book will be a start to helping many children homeopathically, wherever they are on the autism spectrum, to live lives of greater self-fulfilment.

GLOSSARY OF
HOMEOPATHIC TERMS

AGGRAVATION

There may be an intensification of existing symptoms on first taking a homeopathic remedy or a temporary return of old symptoms. This is often a good sign as it shows that the remedy closely matches the patient, any troublesome or long lasting aggravation can be easily managed by a well-trained homeopathic practitioner. An aggravation could also be seen as a 'healing crisis' or 'detox'. Homeopaths expect that symptoms will move from more important to less important organs (from inner to outer), from above downwards, and in reverse order of appearance; this is known as 'Hering's law of cure'.

ALLOPATHY/CONVENTIONAL MEDICINE

Conventional allopathic medicine is based on the principle of treating symptoms with their opposite. For example for nausea an anti-emetic would be prescribed. This is in contrast to homeopathy which is based on the principle of treating 'like with like'.

CEASE THERAPY

CEASE stands for Complete Elimination of Autism Spectrum Expression, a branch of homeopathy developed by Tinus Smits MD.

CLASSICAL HOMEOPATHY

This was developed by Samuel Hahnemann between 1810 and 1842. It is based on the principle of treating 'like with like'. Major proponents of classical homeopathy have been James Tyler Kent, George Vithoulkas and Rajan Sankaran.

COMPLEX HOMEOPATHY

This is when a mixture of potentised medicines is prescribed for a condition. This does not follow the principles of homeopathy, matching the remedy to the individual patient, and is generally not approved of by professionally qualified homeopaths.

DOCTRINE OF SIGNATURES

This concept states that if something, usually a herb, looks like something it will be good to treat that. This can often be seen in the names of plants, for example Lungwort (*Pulmonaria*) was traditionally used as a herb to treat lung problems or Eyebright (*Euphrasia*) to treat eye problems. This concept has little to do with homeopathy, as the information about homeopathic remedies is determined from provings, toxicology reports and clinical experience. Homeopathy works on the inner dynamic or vital force or chi, to use an acupuncture term and views the person as a whole rather than treating individual parts; although organ-specific remedies are used sometimes.

HOMEOPATHY OR HOMOEOPATHY

Homoeopathy is Greek for 'similar suffering' and was the original name given to this system of medicine by its founder. Homeopathy is an Americanisation of the word and has been adopted on the internet, so is now replacing the former, but you may still come across the old form of the word.

ISODE

A potentised preparation of diseased tissue or disease product from the patient themselves.

ISOPATHY/ISOPATHIC REMEDY

An isopathic remedy is a potentised remedy that is prepared from the substance which is postulated to be implicated in the patient's current symptom picture. It could be a nosode, a potentised allopathic drug or a vaccine. The rationale behind the prescription is to act as an antidote based upon the principle of 'never been well since'.

LAW OF SIMILARS

Similia similibus curantur, 'like is cured by like'. A substance which when given to healthy subjects, either in a proving or from accidental toxicological exposure, causes symptoms to occur which are curative when given to sick persons exhibiting similar symptoms. The selection of a remedy is given according to degree of similarity and may be something that the person has never encountered or been exposed to. Isopathic remedies are a substance to which the person has been exposed – and they have never been well since.

MAINTAINING CAUSES OR OBSTACLES TO CURE

Those factors in a person's lifestyle which may contribute to their ongoing ill health. This could be an ongoing emotional stress such as poor relationship with a spouse, boss or parent; continuing exposure to toxic chemicals or to aggravating foods (although it would be hoped that homeopathy would reduce food sensitivities over time), generally poor diet and living conditions. However, the maintaining causes are also influenced by the individual's susceptibility and miasmatic inheritance; to discuss the interplay of all of these factors would be a chapter in itself!

MATERIA MEDICA

A text book listing homeopathic remedies, their sources, mode of preparation and detailed indications for their use. The information about the remedies will be derived from provings upon healthy volunteers, clinical observation and toxicology reports.

MIASMATIC THEORY OR MIASMS

Even before the theory of genetics, homeopaths took into account the influence of heredity on a person's health. The homeopath will commonly ask about the patient's family history and this may influence the choice of remedy. The main miasms are Psora (underfunction), Sycosis (overproduction) and Syphilitic (destructive processes). If there has been a marked family history of tuberculosis, the Tubercular miasm may be seen to be active in a case; if there has been a marked family history of cancer/diabetes/suppression of the inflammatory process the Cancer miasm may be indicated. Obviously we have almost all been exposed to all of these hereditary influences, so it is for the homeopath to determine which is the most active miasm currently.

The nosode of the disease may be prescribed or a remedy which is associated with that particular miasm, hence the frequent prescriptions of remedies such as *Medorrhinum*, key remedy of the sycotic miasm; *Carcinosin*, key remedy of the Cancer miasm; *Mercurius*, key remedy of the Syphilitic miasm; and *Tuberculinum*, key remedy of the Tubercular miasm, for so many children on the autism spectrum.

MODALITIES

Factors which make a condition or a person in general feel better or worse. For example whether a sore throat is better for hot or cold drinks; or whether someone's mood is better or worse at a certain time of day; or whether a child prefers to sleep with the covers on or off.

NEVER BEEN WELL SINCE (NBWS)

If there is an obvious chronological point since when a person's health has declined, this is referred to as NBWS. The homeopath might, if for example a child's health declined after a particular immunisation, either give that vaccine in homeopathic form or prescribe on the overall symptom picture. I have had success with both approaches and sometimes the sequencing of remedies will need to be adjusted according to the particular case.

NOSODE

A potentised preparation of diseased tissue or disease product.

POTENTISATION

Potentisation is the process through which a substance is made into a homeopathic remedy. Homeopathic remedies are made through a process of serial shaking, sucussion and dilution.

PROVING

Provings are referred to frequently in the book: when a new substance is being considered as a homeopathic remedy a 'proving' takes place. A group of 10–30 participants are selected with relatively good health; their baseline health is noted before the start of the proving. They are given the new remedy to take on a trial basis and asked to observe and note down any changes that they experience on taking the remedy, they will also be partnered with a supervisor who they will speak with each day. The proving usually lasts 30 days and at the end of it the participants meet up and compare symptoms experienced. Ideally only the 'master prover' knows what substance is being proved and a number of participants are prescribed placebo. The material is then collated and published.

REPERTORY

The homeopathic repertory is a book or computer software program in which the collated symptoms of each homeopathic remedy are listed under the symptoms which they have produced in provings or clinical practice. It is laid out in a particular format so as to be consistent worldwide.

RUBRICS

A rubric is a list of indicated remedies for a symptom collated from homeopathic provings and clinical experience. The reference book which contains rubrics is known as a 'Repertory', there are both published books and homeopathic software programs with this information.

SIMILIMUM

The homeopathic remedy that most closely matches the symptoms of the patient.

SUSCEPTIBILITY

At any one time an individual's susceptibility to disease will vary, as will their susceptibility in comparison to other people over time. Why is it that one person will catch a cold and not another, or one person catch a contagious skin condition and not another? Each individual has their own makeup consisting of inherited factors, genetics, miasms and exposure to stress both emotional and physical; all of these factors, and more, determine whether you will catch something or not.

VITAL FORCE

Homeopathy is a 'vitalistic' medicine, viewing the body not as a series of mechanical parts but as a whole self-balancing system, the sum of the body is more than its parts. Disease is seen as a dynamic disturbance of the body/mind in totality. Homeopathic remedies are also believed to work on this dynamic level. The 'vital force' is similar to the principle of 'chi' in Chinese medicine.

HOMEOPATHIC ORGANISATIONS

AUSTRALIA
Australian Homeopathic Association
PO Box 7108
Qld 4350
Toowoomba South
Tel: 07 4636 5081
Email: admin@homeopathyoz.org

CANADA
North American Society of Homeopaths
Canada Office
6254 134A Street
Surrey
BC V3X 1K1

Canadian Society of Homeopaths
101–1001 West Broadway
Unit 120
Vancouver
BC V6H 4E4
Tel: 604 803 9242
Email: homeopathy@csoh.ca

UNITED KINGDOM
Alliance of Registered Homeopaths
Millbrook
Millbrook Hill
Nutley
East Sussex

TN22 3PJ
Tel: 01825 714 506
Email: info@a-r-h.org

British Homeopathic Association and Faculty of Homeopathy
Hahnemann House
29 Park Street West
Luton
LU1 3BE
Tel: 01582 408 675
Email: info@britishhomeopathic.org

The Society of Homeopaths
11 Brookfield
Duncan Close
Northampton
NN3 6WL
Tel: 01604 817 890
Email: info@homeopathy-soh.org

USA
Council for Homeopathic Certification
PMB 187
16915 SE 272nd Street
Suite #100
Covington
WA 98042
Tel (toll free): 001 866 242 3399

North American Society of Homeopaths
US Office
PO Box 115
Troy
ME 04987
Tel: 001 206 720 7000
Email: office@homeopathy.org or nashinfo@homeopathy.org

CONTRIBUTORS

MIKE ANDREWS *DSH RSHom*
Tel: 01588 660 793
Email: mike@mikeandrewshomeopathy.co.uk
Website: www.mikeandrewshomeopathy.co.uk

CAROL BOYCE
Email: carol@somethingtosayproductions.com

PHILIPPA FIBERT *BEd (hons cantab), BSc, MSc, RSHom*
The Coppins
Horsleys Green
High Wycombe
Bucks
HP14 3UX
UK
Tel: 07543 345 046
Email: philippahomeopath@hotmail.co.uk

LINLEE JORDAN *Dip Hom Dip Nut RN Masters Health Sc Ed*
Harbord Homeopathic Children's Clinic
110/20 Dale Street
Brookvale
NSW 2100
Australia
Tel: 02 990 59415
Email: info@hhcc.com.au

DR. M.A. RAJALAKSHMI
1080
12th Main
West of Chord Road 2nd Stage
Rajajinagar
Bangalore 560086 India
Tel (mobile): ++91 9449 163 350
Website: sites.google.com/site/anjanahomeocare
Email: homeodr.raji@gmail.com

DANNY DUSHAN RON
Email: danny@adivclassic.co.il
Website: www.adivclassic.co.il

FRAN SHEFFIELD *Postgraduate Hon Studies*
RN RM Masters Health Sc Ed AHA AROH
7B
1 Pioneer
Tuggerah 2259
New South Wales
Australia
Tel: +612 4304 0822
Email: office@homeopathyplus.co.au
Website: www.homeopathyplus.com.au

SIMON TAFFLER *PCH RSHom FSHom*
Tel: London 07967 645 960; New York 001 212 560 5661

REFERENCES

Allen, T.F. (1990) *The Encyclopaedia of Pure Materia Medica Volume 2*. New Delhi: Jain Publishers.

American Psychiatric Association (2013) 'DSM-5 Autism Spectrum Disorder Fact Sheet.' *Diagnostic and Statistical Manual of Mental Disorders V*. Washington, DC: American Psychiatric Association. Available at http://www.psychiatry.org/dsm5, accessed on 20 May 2014.

Attwood, T. (2003) *Asperger's Syndrome DVD*. London: Jessica Kingsley Publishers.

AutismOne (2013) *About Us – Autism Spectrum Disorder*. Autism International Association, Inc. Available at www.autismone.org/content/about-us, accessed on 23 December 2013.

Autism Spectrum Australia (2013) *What is Autism?* Available at www.aspect.org.au/content/what-autism, accessed on 20 March 2014.

Autistic UK (2014) 'Home page.' North Shields UK. Available at http:// autisticuk.org/, accessed 21 March 2014.

Barron, P. and Jordan, L. (2009) 'Hyoscyamus: A case series analysis.' *Similia: The Australian Journal of Homeopathic Medicine, 21*, 1, 34–38.

Barvalia, P. (2011) 'Autism spectrum disorder: holistic homeopathy part one.' *Homeopathic Links, 24*, 31–38.

Benveniste, J., Davenas, E., Ducot, B. *et al.* (1991) L'agitation de Solutions Hautement Diluées n'induit pas d'activité Biologique Specifique. *Comptes Rendus de l'Académie des Sciences*, 312, 461–466.

Borg, T., (2013) *Commissioner Borg addresses the European Parliament's Interest Group on Complementary and Alternative Medicine*. European Parliament. Available at http://ec.europa.eu/commission_2010-2014/borg/docs/speech_cancer_27062013_en.pdf, accessed on 24 January 2013.

Bornhöft, G., and Matthiessen, P. (eds) (2012) *Homeopathy in Healthcare Effectiveness, Appropriateness, Safety, Costs*. Abstract. Springer Publications worldwide. Available at http://www.springer.com/medicine/complementary+%26+alternative+medicine/book/978-3-642-20637-5, accessed 21 March 2014.

British Broadcasting Corporation (2009) *Horizon*. Ghost genes. Available at http://www.bbc.co.uk/sn/tvradio/programmes/horizon/ghostgenes.shtml, accessed on 21 November 2013.

Boyce, C. (2010) 'Lost generation: the rise and rise of regressive autism.' *Homeopathy in Practice*, Autumn, 16–19.

Boyce, C. (2013) 'Saving a lost generation.' Something to Say Productions. Available at www.savingalostgeneration.com, accessed 23 September 2013.

Bradford (2013) 'CDC study debunks autism - vaccine link.' *Passport Health Baltimore*. Available at http://www.passporthealthusa.com/2013/04/cdc-study-debunks-vaccine-autism-link, accessed 18 March 2014.

Centre for Academic Primary Care (2013) 'Welcome to MYMOP.' Available at www.bms.ac.uk/primaryhealthcare/resources/mymop/, accessed 7 May 2014.

Dante's mom (2012) 'Helium rocks (June 24th 2012).' *Boy Connected: Improving Dante's health and wellbeing using the CEASE homeopathic protocol along with others.* Blog available at http://boyconnected.blogspot.co.uk/2012/06/helium-rocks.html, accessed 30 November 2013.

Elia, K. (2012) *Materia Medica of Autism Parts 1 and 2.* USA broadcast. Available at www.wholehealthnow/courses.com, accessed 30 November 2013.

Emam, A.M., Esmat, M.M. and Sadex, A.A. (2012) '*Candida albicans* infection in autism.' *Journal of American Science, 8,* 12.

Emanuele, E., Colombo, R., Martinelli, V., Brondino, N., Marini, M., Boso M., Barale F. and Politi, P. (2010) 'Elevated urine levels of bufotenine in patients with autistic spectrum disorders and schizophrenia.' *Neuro Endocrinology Letters, 31,* 1, 117–21. Available at www.unboundmedicine.com/medline/citation/20150873/Elevated_urine_levels_of_bufotenine_in_patients_with_autistic_spectrum_disorders_and_schizophrenia_, accessed 24 January 2014.

European Parliament (1996) *Charter of Rights for persons with Autism.* Quoted at http://www.autismeurope.org/publications/rights-and-autism-2/charter-of-rights-4/?page=2, accessed 24 January 2014.

Feingold Association of the United States (2014) *Symptoms that may be helped by the Feingold Program.* Fishers, Indiana: Feingold Association of the United States. Available at http://www.feingold.org/symptoms.php, accessed 22 May 2014.

Fibert, P. (2012) 'Nature or nurture: what drives the rise in behavioural disorders?' *The Homeopath, 30,* 4, 15–17.

Find a Homeopath (2013) *Team GB sprinter James Ellington says... homeopathy works* findahomeopath.org.uk.

Fontaine, P. (2012) *Reversing Autism with Classic Homeopathy.* New York: Homeopathic Services Inc. Available at http://homeopathicservices.com/blog/reversing-autism-with-classic-homeopathy/, accessed 30 July 2013.

Gamble, J. (2010) *Mastering Homeopathy 3 – Obstacles to Cure: Toxicity, Deficiency and Infection.* Sydney: Karuna Health Care Publishing.

Geier, D.A. and Geier, M.R. (2006) 'Early downward trends in neurodevelopmental disorders following removal of thimerosal-containing vaccines.' *Journal of American Physicians and Surgeons, 11,* 1, 8–13.

Grandin, T. and Johnson, C. (2005) *Animals in Translation: Using the Mysteries of Autism to Decode Animal Behaviour.* London and New York: Bloomsbury.

Gupta, N., Saxena, R.K, Malhotra, A.K. and Juneja, R. (2010) 'Homoeopathic medicinal treatment of autism.' *Indian Journal of Research in Homoeopathy, 4,* 4, 19–28.

Hahnemann, S. (1842) (translated by W. Boericke 1921) *The Organon of Medicine 6th Edition.* New Delhi: Homeopathic Publications.

Hahnemann, S. (1842) (translated by W.B. O'Reilly 1996) *The Organon of the Medical Art.* Redmond, WA, Birdcage Books.

Halladay, A. (2013) 'Autism and infertility treatment: your questions answered.' *Autism Speaks,* available at http://www.autismspeaks.org/science/science-news/autism-and-infertility-treatment-yourquestions-answered, accessed 27 March 2014.

Hartmann, F. (1998) *The Life and Doctrines of Paracelsus.* Pomeroy: Health Research Books.

Herscu, P. (2010) *Homeopathic Treatment of Autism – Putting the Pieces Together.* Kandern: Narayana Publishers.

Hickman, M.A., Zeng, C., Farche, A. *et al.* (2013) '*Candida albicans* forms mating competent haploids.' *Nature, 494,* 7435, 55–59.

Jordan, L. (2012) *Challenging Children: Success with Homeopathy Second Edition.* Kandern: Narayana Publishers.

Kaiser, B. and Rasminsky, J. (2012) *Challenging Behaviour in Young Children: Understanding, Preventing, and Responding Effectively,* 3rd edition. Upper Saddle River, NJ: Pearson Education.

Kim, Y.S. (2011) 'Prevalence of autism spectrum disorders in a total population sample.' *The American Journal of Psychiatry, 168, 9*, 904–12. Abstract available at http://www.ncbi.nlm. nih.gov/pubmed/21558103, accessed 6 December 2013.

Kirk, S. (2010) *Hope for the Autism Spectrum.* London and Philadelphia: Jessica Kingsley Publishers.

Lansky, A. (2003) *Impossible Cure: The Promise of Homeopathy.* Portola Valley, CA: Ranch Press.

Lansky, A. (2005) *Interview with Nancy Frederick.* Podcast available at http://www.autismone. org/content/interview-homeopath-nancy-frederick, accessed 12 November 2013.

Lansky, A., (2012) *Max's Story – A Homeopathic Cure of Autism.* Available at www.homeopathysnc.org/ autism_recovery_amy_lansky.htm, accessed 7 May 2014.

Latchis, S. (2001) *Homeopathy and Autism – Review.* New England: New England School of Homeopathy. Available at www.nesh.com/course-seminar-offerings/course-and-seminar-reviews/homeopathy-and-autism/, accessed 30 November 2013.

Macedo de Menezes Fonseca, G.R., de Almeida Bolognani, F., Ferreira Duras, F., Maio Souza, K. *et al.* (2008) 'Effect of homeopathic medication on the cognitive and motor performance of autistic children (Pilot study).' *International Journal of High Dilution Research, 7,* 23, 63–71.

Markram, K., Rinaldi, T., La Mendola, D., Sandi, C. and Markram, H. (2008) 'Abnormal fear conditioning and amygdala processing in animal model of autism.' *Neuropsychopharmacology, 33,* 901–912.

Master, F. (2002) *State of Mind Influencing the Foetus.* New Delhi: B. Jain Publishers.

Master, F. (2006) *Clinical Observations of Children's Remedies,* 3rd edition. Eindhoven: Lutra.

McNeill, F. (2011) 'Small Remedies, Big Results'. *Autism Eye,* Issue 4 Winter 2011/12, 22–24.

Maeseneer, J.M de., Drie, M.L. van, Green, L.A. and Weel, C. van (2003) 'The need for research in primary care.' *Lancet, 362,* 932, 1314–1320.

Montagnier, L., Aïssa, J., Ferris, S., Montagnier, J.-L. and Lavallée, C. (2009) 'Electromagnetic signals are produced by aqueous nanostructures derived from bacterial DNA sequences.' *Interdisciplinary Sciences: Computatiorial Life Sciences, 1,* 81–90.

Montagnier, L. (2010) 'Speech to the Lindau Nobel Laureate Meeting, 28 June 2010', Lindau Nobel Laureate Meeting, Lindau, Germany.

Montagnier, L., Aïssa, J., Del Giuduice, E., Lavallée, C., Tedeschi, A. and Vitiello, G. (2011) 'DNA waves and water.' *Journal of Physics Conference Series, 306.*

Ozonoff, S. Heung, K. Byrd, R., Hansen, R. and Hertz-Picciotto, I. (2008) 'The onset of autism: Patterns of symptom emergence in the first years of life.' *Autism Research, 1,* 6, 320–328.

Petrucci, R. (2009) *Homeopathic Treatment of Children Seminar,* 23–24 May 2009, London, seminar notes by Andrews, M.

Rajalakshmi, M.A. (2007) 'Role of homoeopathy in the management of autism: Study of effects of homoeopathic treatment on the autism triad.' *Internet Journal of Alternative Medicine, 6,* 1. Available at http://ispub.com/IJAM/7/2/8801, accessed December 2013.

Reichenberg-Ullman, J., Ullman, R. and Luepker, I. (2005) *A Drug-Free Approach to Asperger Syndrome and Autism: Homeopathic Care for Exceptional Kids.* Edmonds, WA: Picnic Point Press.

Research Autism (2013) *Autism: Treatments, Therapies, Interventions.* London: Research Autism. Available at http://researchautism.net/pages/autism_treatments_therapies_interventions/autismtreatment_introduction, accessed 21 October 2013.

Rhijn, A. van (2011) 'A three stage approach.' *Homeopathic Links, 24,* 97–105.

Rimland, B. and Edelson, S. (1999) *Autism Treatment Evaluation Check-list.* San Diego, CA: Autism Research Institute. Available at www.surveygizmo.com/s3/1329619/Autism-Treatment-Evaluation-Checklist-revised, accessed 17 January 2014.

Ron, D. (2013) 'Candida mix: A case study and information about Candidemia.' *Similia, 25,*1, 12–14.

Ronald, A. Pennell, C. and Whitehouse, A. (2010) 'Prenatal maternal stress associated with ADHD and autistic traits in early childhood.' *Frontiers in Psychology, 1,* 223, 1–8.

Rothenberg, A. (2010) 'Special kids, special care.' *Spectrum of Homeopathy, 1 (Childhood and Psyche)*, 56–60.

Schlepper, L. (2011) *Homeopathy for Autism: How to take Remedies.* App. Palo Alto, CA: Arende Inc. Available at http://www.aerende.com/index.html, accessed 27 March 2014.

Schepper, L. (2013) 'ASD and Homeopathic Intervention.' Available at http://www.drluc.com/ASDHomeopathic.asp, accessed 21 November 2013.

Scholten, J. (2010) 'Overcoming the false self.' *Spectrum of Homeopathy (Childhood and Psyche)*, 1 2010, 22–26. Kandern: Narayana Publishers.

Scholten, J. (1996) *Homoeopathy and the Elements.* Utrecht: Stichting Alonnissos.

Schubert, C. (2010) 'New Psycho-epidemics'. *Spectrum of Homeopathy (Childhood and Psyche)*, 1 2010, 4–7. Kander: Narayana Publishers.

Schroyens, F. and Hamilton, I. (2012) 'Collaborations: an interview with Frederik Schroyens.' *The Homeopath (Childhood and Psyche)*, *31*, 2, 3–6.

Schroyens, F. (2013) *Synthesis 10.5 Treasure Edition repertory.* Available at http://www.archibd.com/radar10.html, accessed 30 November 2013.

Shattock, P., Waltz, M. and Whiteley P., (2004) 'The use of medication for people with autism spectrum disorders.' Paper presented at Autism Research Institute Durham Conference. Available at www.espa-research.org.uk/linked/medication.pdf, accessed 4 December 2013.

Sheffield, F. (2008) 'Homoeopathy and the treatment of autism spectrum disorders (part two)' *Similia, 20, 1*, 11–30.

Sinclair, J. (1993) 'Don't Mourn for Us.' *Our Voice, 1*, 3. Available at www.autreat.can/dont_mourn.html, accessed 21 March 2014.

Smits, T., 2010 *Autism Beyond Despair – Cease Therapy. Homeopathy has the Answers.* Haarlem, Emryss Publishers

Theoharides, T. Asadi, S. and Patel, A. (2013) 'Focal brain inflammation and autism.' *Journal of Neuroinflammation, 10*, 46, 1–7.

Tiller, W. (1981) Foreword in G. Vithoulkas (1986) *The Science of Homeopathy.* London: Thorsons Publishing Group.

Vermeulen, F. (2004) *Prisma: The Arcana of Materia Medica Illuminated. Similars and Parallels Between Substance and Remedy,* 3rd edition. Haarlem: Emryss Publishers.

Vithoulkas, G. (1986) *The Science of Homeopathy.* London: Thorsons Publishing Group.

Weiland, J. (2010) 'Pathway into Life'. *Spectrum Homeopathy, (Childhood and Psyche)*, 1 2010, 8–13. Kandern: Narayana Publishers.

Welte, U. (2010) *Colors in Homeopathy Textbook: Color Repertory with Instructions.* Kandern: Narayana Publishers.

Welte, U. and Kuntosch, M. (2010) 'Shy, odd, really brainy. Lithium and Lanthanides in the autism spectrum – a practical differential diagnosis.' *Spectrum of Homeopathy (Childhood and Psyche)* 01/2010. Kandern: Narayana Publishers.

Whiteley, P. and Shattock, P. (2002) 'Biochemical aspects in autism spectrum disorders: Updating the opioid-excess theory and presenting new opportunities for biomedical intervention.' *Expert Opinions of Therapeutic Targets, 6*, 175–83. Available at www.ncbi.nlm.nih.gov/pubmed/12223079, accessed 4 December 2013.

Whiteley, P., Rodgers, J., Savery, D. and Shattock, P. (1999) 'A gluten-free diet as an intervention for autism and associated spectrum disorders: Preliminary findings.' *Autism, 3,1*, 45–65.

World Health Organization (2005) 'Status of homeopathy worldwide.' Available at http://drnancymalik.wordpress.com/article/status-of-homeopathy/, accessed 6 December 2013.

Yehuda, R., Mulherin Engel, S., Brand, S.R., Seckl, J., Marcus, S.M. and Berkowitz, G.S. (2005) 'Transgenerational effects of posttraumatic stress disorder in babies of mothers exposed to the World Trade Centre attacks during pregnancy.' *Journal of Clinical Endocrinology and Metabolism.* Available at http://jcem.endojournals.org/content/90/7/4115.full, accessed 17 January 2014.

Yui, T. and Hamilton, I. (2011) 'The East Japan earthquake.' *The Homeopath, 30*, 3, 24.

SUBJECT INDEX

AUTHOR INDEX